Herbs For Healing
101 Herbal Remedies
What Are They
What Are They Used For

Also By Brian B Jacques

His very popular Series of Mini-Health Books includes:

- An Easy Way To Understand Eczema and Psoriasis
- An Easy Way To Understand Stress and Depression
- An Easy Way To Understand Vitamins and Minerals
- An Easy Way To Understand Parasites, Worms, Candida, Constipation & Detoxing
- An Easy Way To Understand Crohn's Disease and IBD
- An Easy Way To Understand Body Building For Men And Women
- An Easy Way To Understand Alzheimer's Disease
- An Easy Way To Understand Herpes
- An Easy Way To Understand Parkinson's Disease
- An Easy Way To Understand Autism
- An Easy Way To Understand Fibromyalgia
- An Easy Way To Understand Your Body Systems
- An Easy Way To Understand Erectile Dysfunction
- An Easy Way To Understand Heart Disease, High Blood Pressure & Stroke
- An Easy Way To Understand Detoxing For Men & Women
- How To Lose Weight After 40
- How To Lose Weight And Maintain Your Ideal Weight Permanently
- Amino Acids & Enzymes—What Are They & Why Do You Need Them
- The Little A–Z Dictionary of Herbal Remedies
- The Magic Of Vitamins & Minerals
- Effective Methods To Stop Smoking

All these books are available as Kindle Editions (available from the Kindle Store on Amazon.com, and other countries Amazon sites where the Kindle platform is supported.) Many of these books are also available for the Barnes and Noble "Nook". In addition, all these titles will shortly be available as print editions from the Amazon website. A downloadable eBook version will also be available from the publishers website at www.wisdomforlifemedia.com

Herbs For Healing
101 Herbal Remedies
What Are They
What Are They Used For

Brian B Jacques

Wisdom For Life Media

Publisher: Wisdom For Life Media (www.wisdomforlifemedia.com)

While they have made every effort to verify the information provided in this publication, neither the author nor the publisher assumes any responsibility for errors in, omissions from, or different interpretation of the subject matter.

The information herein may be subject to varying laws, regulations, and practices in different areas, states and countries. The purchaser or reader assumes all responsibility for use of the information.

All information included within this book is for educational purposes only. The author and publishers do not attempt to diagnose or treat any medical conditions, be it to do with health, diet or exercise.

If you consider that you have any kind of medical condition, then, you should consult a qualified medical practitioner or doctor or qualified naturopathic doctor before starting any herbal, vitamin and/or mineral program or supplement regime, exercise or health training program or diet suggested in this book.

This book is not intended for anyone under the age of 18 years, nor is it intended for breast feeding or pregnant women, underweight people or anyone with eating disorders or a health condition that requires special diets or medical treatment.

The author and publishers disclaim any liability for any loss however caused by anyone using the information contained in this book.

Images

All images are either copyright the author, or are used under the terms of a Royalty Free License.

ISBN - 13: 978-1503075047

ISBN - 10: 1503075044

Published in The United States of America

"Education is the kindling of a flame, not the filling of a vessel." —Socrates

Contents

Also By Brian B Jacques..2

Acknowledgment...9

Herbs – An Ancient, Natural Medicinal Treatment 11

Do You Live In a European Union Country? 15

An A to Z of Herbs..17

Consult Your Doctor or a Naturopathic Doctor 125

About The Author 126

Would You Like a Reliable Supplier of Natural Vitamins, Minerals and Herbal Products?...127

Index of Health Conditions 128

Index of Herbs 142

Acknowledgment

To the many people I have come into contact with throughout my life, whose belief in me has made everything possible and worthwhile.

Herbs – An Ancient, Natural Medicinal Treatment

Herbal medicine is the oldest known form of healthcare. Whether it is Western natural medicine, or Chinese, Indian or Native American, herbal combinations are used to improve the performance of various body organs.

The Chinese emperor Shen Nong (who lived around 5000BC) wrote a treatise on herbs that is still in use today. For example, Shen Nong recommended the use of Ma Huang (known as ephedra in the Western world), to treat respiratory problems. Ephedrine, extracted from ephedra, is used as a decongestant today.

In another example, King Hammurabi of Babylon (c. 1800BC) recommended the use of mint for digestive disorders. Today, peppermint is widely used to relieve nausea—especially travel sickness and vomiting.

The Middle East in particular has a rich history of herbal healing. Surviving texts from the ancient people's of Mesopotamia, Egypt and India explain with words and pictures how to use medicinal plant products, such as castor oil, linseed oil and white poppies.

During the Middle Ages, most households would have an extensive herb garden which was used to treat all the family's ailments. Home grown herbal plants were the only form of medicine available. The medicinal uses for these herbal plants were passed from generation to generation within a family by word of mouth.

In Europe, in 1649, Nicholas Culpeper wrote *A Physical Directory* and a few years later *The English Physician*. This herbal pharmacopeia was one of the first manuals that anyone could use for health care, and it is still often quoted from today.

In the nineteenth century, Western medicine as we know it today, progressed from being passed on from generation to generation where everyone who was interested had medicinal knowledge, to the realm of just a few that had a more scientific background.

This came about by scientific methods being developed to extract and synthesize active ingredients in plants to manufacture drugs. And a huge and powerful drugs industry was born.

Herbal plants contain many different compounds, active ingredients in the form of alkaloids, volatile oils, vitamins, minerals, glycosides, bioflavonoids, and other ingredients that are important in supporting a particular herbs medicinal qualities. Some of these substances have been identified, but many more have yet to be discovered.

The problem that then arises is when drugs are manufactured; an active ingredient is extracted from the natural herb and synthesized in a laboratory to emulate the natural herb's qualities. But all the other ingredients in the plant are left behind. These "other ingredients" play the role of a natural safeguard which is lost.

By comparison, it usually takes a larger amount of a whole herb, with all of its components, to reach a toxic level. The end result with the drug and its isolated active ingredient is that some of these substances can become toxic in small amounts, which can cause serious side effects from the use of these drugs.

Interestingly, watching drug commercials on TV, most of the time is taken up explaining all the side effects which the drug can cause.

Today components from plants form the basis of many medications used for such conditions as asthma, high blood pressure and heart disease to name a few.

Two examples: salicylic acid, a precursor of aspirin, was originally derived from white willow bark and the meadowsweet plant. Digitalis which is derived from the foxglove plant has been used for many years as a heart medication.

Herbs generally fall into two categories: those that grow in the wild and are called wild crafted. These are harvested where the plant grows in its natural habitat. The other is commercially grown, where a greater control over quality and growing conditions can be exercised.

Herbal products are available in several forms: liquid, tablets, capsules, tinctures, teas, salves, ointments, fresh, or as dried plant parts. Some are supplied as single herbs while others are made into combinations to treat a specific condition.

Capsules and Tablets

The herb is ground into a very fine powder and then either inserted into a capsule or pressed into a tablet form. Generally, herbs in capsules and tablets are less potent than tinctures or extracts. Additionally, read the label to make sure no fillers have been added. Fillers could be either natural or synthetic.

Extracts

Extracts can be made with alcohol like tinctures, or glycerin or water can be used. Like tinctures the herb is in a concentrated form and is easily assimilated by the body. The only way to tell what method has been used is to read the label.

Lozenges

Lozenges are often sucked to ward off the effects of a cold or cough, or they may be used as a decongestant. Many are fortified with vitamin C. Read the label to make sure they are not coated with refined sugar or an artificial sweetener.

Ointments, Salves, and Rubs

There are many products available in your health food store or on the Internet to treat burns, wounds, skin rashes and insect bites, or as heat producing herbs to treat sprains, pulled muscles or to relax muscle aches.

Teas

A huge selection of herbal teas is available either from your health food store, supermarket or on the Internet. Herbal teas take several forms from being relaxing, comforting or having medicinal properties. They come either as loose tea or in tea bags. Either way, they just need preparing with hot water for a very beneficial drink.

Tinctures

A tincture usually contains alcohol which is used to extract and concentrate the active properties of the herb. Tinctures are very easily assimilated by the body and are therefore a very easy and effective way to take a herbal product. If you wish to lessen the effect of the alcohol, then pour the tincture into a small amount of very hot water for a few minutes. The alcohol will vaporize and after it has cooled, it will be ready to drink.

Herbal products, unlike drugs, will take time to provide a beneficial effect in the body. The time scale could be a few weeks to a few months, depending on what the herbal preparation is being used for.

The reason for this is that in some cases, but not all, the herb will supply various "actions" in the body. First a cleansing or neutralizing action; next possibly an antiseptic action, followed by a deodorizing action, and finally a building action to re-build the body back to full health. As you can appreciate, all this takes time, but it is well worth the wait in the long run.

The quality of the raw material used will determine the potency of the finished herbal product. Therefore it is well worth while doing a little research on a particular supplier or manufacturer before you part with your money.

Although the title of this book is Herbs For Healing, you will notice that I have also included a few plants (and trees) which contain beneficial compounds that can be beneficial for maintaining your good health, such as Papaya, Psyllium. and Pygeum.

Do You Live In a European Union Country?

Of particular concern in Europe. In 2011 the European Union introduced the Herbal Medicines Directive which means the herbal industry has been all but destroyed by a draconian law which has virtually banned the supply of herbal products within the European Union.

The excuse for issuing this directive is "to ensure public safety with regard to herbal products". I would have thought that something that has been used safely for hundreds (and in some cases thousands) of years would be safe for the public to take.

Many herbal products have been classified, not for use in food preparation (i.e. for cooking or garnishing purposes) but as "medicines" and a company now needs a license in order to sell them to the public. The cost of the license is in the order of $150,000 per herbal product. Yes, you read that correctly, $150,000 per herbal product.

Say you are a manufacturer and have just a small range of just 20 herbal products, that is going to cost you $3,000,000 in license fees, before you can sell anything. Very few manufacturers have that kind of money to waste on licenses for something that has been used safely for all those years.

All this new law is going to do is drive the supply of these safe, natural herbal products underground. With the power of modern communications and the Internet, all you have to do is spend a little time seeking out those herbal products you require from sources outside Europe. Many suppliers in other parts of the world—and especially the United States—will be more than happy to supply you, and will ship their products internationally. As the saying goes—where there's a will there's a way!!

When buying any herbal product, make sure there are no artificial fillers, binders or artificial sugar coatings. Tablets can contain magnesium stearate or stearic acid which is used as a lubricant in the manufacturing process. Binders can be added to help hold the ingredients together. Often artificial colors are added to make the product look good. A shellac coating can be added which will be listed in the ingredients as "natural glaze." Capsules can have fillers added to fill-up the capsule.

Only buy natural herbal products—not synthetic ones. Make sure you do your research on the supplier / manufacturer before purchasing.

An A to Z of Herbs

Alfalfa

Plant Parts Used Leaves

Alfalfa is a grass which contains all the essential amino acids as well as being rich in trace minerals and enzymes. It assists in the assimilation of protein, calcium and other nutrients. Alfalfa contains chlorophyll; therefore it is an excellent body cleanser, natural deodorizer and infection fighter. It is frequently taken to lessen the effects of hay fever allergies. It is also fed to horses as a counter to arthritic conditions and digestive problems.

As it is a good source of fiber, it is useful for detoxifying the body in addition to improving liver health.

Alfalfa contains vitamin A, D, K, and minerals calcium, iron, phosphorus, iron and potassium, in addition to various enzymes.

Historical uses:	
Allergies (Various)	Anemia
Arthritis	Bad Breath
Blood Purifier	Bowel Problems
Bursitis	Cholesterol Reduction
Cleanses the Kidneys	Digestive System Disorders
High Blood Pressure	Mental and Physical Fatigue
Mild Diuretic	Pituitary Gland Support
Reduces Fever	Stimulates Appetite
Tonic	Urinary System Disorders

Barberry

Plant Parts Used: Bark

Barberry has been valued for its antibiotic action for over 2,000 years. The active ingredient in Barberry—Berberine is a very potent fighter against bacterial infections. In addition it also stimulates the immune system and assists in reducing high blood pressure due to its ability to dilate blood vessels.

It has a very positive action on the liver—assisting in the flow of bile which is important in all liver conditions, but especially jaundice.

Barberry contains vitamin C and minerals iron, magnesium and phosphorus.

Historical Uses:	
Bacterial Infections	Blood Purifier
Fever	Gall Bladder Problems
Gas	High Blood Pressure
Indigestion	Jaundice
Liver Conditions	Nervous System Disorders

Basil

Plant Parts Used: Leaves and Tops of Flowers

Basil is often thought of as a culinary product—especially for use in pasta sauce. However, it has been used for thousands of years to treat a variety of ailments including intestinal parasites and worms as well as being an excellent treatment for other intestinal conditions.

Indian researchers have also used Basil Oil successfully to treat various skin infections such as acne.

Basil is also useful in drawing out poisons from wasp and hornet stings as well as the venom from snake bites.

As it is an excellent antispasmodic, it is also helpful in cases of whooping cough

Basil contains vitamin A, B2 (Riboflavin), D, and minerals calcium, iron, magnesium and phosphorus.

Historical Uses:	
Acne	Colds
Fever	Flu
Headaches	Indigestion
Insect Bites	Parasites
Respiratory Infections	Snake Bites
Whooping Cough	Worms

Bayberry

Plant Parts Used: Bark

Used by early American settlers for a variety of conditions including: colds and flu when combined with ginger or capsicum. The root bark contains an antibiotic chemical called myricitrin which has the ability to combat various bacteria strains as well as protozoa.

Myricitrin also play a key role in alleviating the effects of diarrhea and dysentery, in addition to reducing the effects of fever.

Bayberry also supports the adrenal glands as well as being a blood cleanser and removing waste material from arteries and veins.

Bayberry contains vitamin C.

Historical Uses:	
Adrenal Gland Support	Blood Cleanser
Catarrh	Colds
Diarrhea	Dysentery
Fever	Flu
Glandular System Support	Liver Conditions
Parasites	Sore Throat

Bilberry

Plant Parts Used: Fruit

Bilberry and its close cousin blueberry are often confused as they each have a dark blue smooth skin. Bilberry has been used for medicinal purposes in Europe since the 16th century. By comparison, blueberry has been widely cultivated in the US since the 1920s. They are both potent antioxidants and are therefore excellent free radial scavengers.

Bilberry (and blueberry) is often associated with providing benefits for eye vision. This was apparent during World War 11 when bomber pilots flying night bombing missions over occupied Europe found that their night vision improved if they ate bilberry jam before leaving on their missions.

Bilberry strengthens the tiny capillaries that surround the eyes. In so doing, it improves circulation and thus increases the ability of fluids and nutrients to more easily pass through.

However, eye vision is not the only benefits derived from bilberry. Bilberry is excellent for supporting the entire circulatory system. It improves circulation to the hands, feet, brain and heart. The incidence of blood clots can be reduced as well as reducing the risk of atherosclerosis.

By combining bilberry with vitamin E, the formation of cataracts can be reduced; it also has the ability to protect the eyes from the effects of diabetes.

Bilberry contains minerals calcium, iron, magnesium, manganese, phosphorus, potassium, selenium, silicon, sodium and zinc. It is also an excellent source of beneficial bioflavonoids.

Historical Uses:	
Blood Thinner	Blood Vessels
Circulatory System Support	Cold Hands and Feet
Diarrhea	Kidney Problems
Night Blindness	Raynaud's Disease
Sensitivity to Light	Supports the Immune System
Varicose Veins	

Blackberry

Plant Parts Used: Leaves, Bark, Roots and Fruit

Blackberry is often associated with jam or is often eaten as berries. However, it has tremendous medicinal properties.

Because it has a high tannin content—which makes it more astringent—this makes it an excellent treatment for diarrhea and dysentery. This astringent action also makes it useful in wound healing as it constricts blood vessels and stops minor bleeding.

Eating the berries can help alleviate the effects of mouth sores as well as the effects of a sore throat. And finally, it has uses as a treatment for hemorrhoids due to its astringent action.

Blackberry contains vitamins A, vitamin B1 (Thiamine), B2 (Riboflavin), B3 (Niacin), C, and minerals calcium and iron.

Historical Uses:	
Bleeding Gums	Diarrhea
Dysentery	Fever
Gargle	Hemorrhoids
Minor Bleeding (Wounds)	Mouth Sores
Sore Throat	Upset Stomach
Wound Healing	

Black Cohosh

Plant Parts Used: Rhizome, Root

Because it contains natural estrogen, Black Cohosh is widely used to treat menopausal symptoms such as hot flashes, night sweats, migraines, mood swings, heart palpitations and dryness. It is also an excellent tonic for the central nervous system.

Black Cohosh contains vitamin A, B8 (Inositol)—although not strictly a B vitamin as it occurs naturally in human cells, B5 (Pantothenic Acid), and minerals phosphorus and silicon.

Historical Uses:	
Balances Hormones	Cramps
Headaches	Heart Stimulant
High Blood Pressure	Hot Flashes
Hysteria	Kidney Problems
Liver Problems	Lungs
Menopause	Menstrual Problems
Nervous Disorders	Pain
Uterine Problems	

Black Walnut

Plant Parts Used: Hulls, Leaves

Traditionally used as a nutritional aid for the intestinal system, Black Walnut has the same laxative action as cascara sagrada, but it works more gently. Due to its astringent qualities, Black Walnut has the power to assist the body in protecting itself from harmful agents such as parasitic worms. It also has the ability to balance blood sugar levels. Black Walnut has a high iodine content, which is good for energy as it supports thyroid function.

Black Walnut contains vitamin B15 (Pangamic Acid) and minerals calcium, iron, magnesium, manganese, phosphorus, potassium and silica. It is also a source of protein

Historical Uses:	
Abscesses	Balances Blood Sugar Levels
Colitis	Constipation
Eye Diseases	Fever
Gargle	Glandular System Support
Hemorrhoids	Infections
Internal Parasites	Laxative
Mouth Sores	Ringworm
Skin Rashes	Thyroid Function
Tonsillitis	Tumors
Worms	Wound Healing

Blessed Thistle

Plant Parts Used: Whole Herb

Blessed Thistle has many uses in the herbal medicine chest. It is a memory booster by supplying oxygen to the brain. It helps reduce fevers. It is a great herb for females in assisting with the effects of menopausal problems. Blessed Thistle also supports the digestive system and is an overall tonic for the body.

Blessed Thistle contains vitamin B Complex and minerals calcium, iron, manganese, phosphorus and potassium.

Historical Uses:	
Balances Hormones	Blood Circulation
Constipation	Cramps
Digestive System Support	Enhances Memory Function
Fever	Gall Bladder Support
Gas	Headaches
Kidneys	Memory
Menstrual Problems	Purifies the Blood
Respiratory infections	Senility
Spleen Support	Strengthens the Heart
Strengthens the Lungs	

Blue Cohosh

Plant Parts Used: Root

Blue Cohosh is not related to Black Cohosh—they originate in different botanical families. Native Americans called Blue Cohosh papoose root thinking that it triggered labor and hastened childbirth.

In addition to its use to induce labor, it has historically also been used to treat cases of arthritis, epilepsy, hiccups, infant colic and sore throat.

As it is an antispasmodic, Blue Cohosh also supports the nervous system. It is especially useful for relieving muscle cramps and spasms.

Blue Cohosh contains vitamin B Complex, E, and minerals calcium, magnesium, phosphorus and potassium.

Historical Uses:	
Arthritis	Bladder infection
Cramps	Colic
Convulsions	Diabetes
Epilepsy	High Blood Pressure
Induces Labor	Inflammation
Regulates Menstruation	Muscle Cramps
Nervous System Support	Neuralgia
Pregnancy disorders	Spasms
Sore Throat	Uterine Problems
Vaginitis	

Blue Vervain

Plant Parts Used: Whole Herb

Blue Vervain is one of the best herbs to take to alleviate the effects of the common cold. For bronchial problems Blue Vervain has the ability to remove phlegm from the chest.

Blue Vervain also supports the nervous system and in this role it acts as a natural tranquilizer and creates a calming and relaxing feeling.

Blue Vervain contains vitamin C, E and minerals calcium and manganese.

Historical Uses:	
Asthma	Bladder Control
Bronchitis	Catarrh
Colds	Colon Health
Consumption	Chest & Throat Congestion
Convulsions	Cough
Earache	Expels Mucus & Phlegm
Headaches	Insomnia
Lowers Fever	Normalizes Bowel Function
Nervous System Support	Tranquilizer

Boneset

Plant Parts Used: Leaves and Flower Tops

Boneset has nothing to do with repairing broken bones!

This herb is an effective treatment for bacterial and viral infections. It achieves this by stimulating the immune system to attack these foreign invaders.

Native Americans introduced Boneset to early colonists as a sweat-inducer to relieve the effects of a fever, such as: influenza, cholera, dengue fever, malaria and typhoid. It was also used to treat an arthritic condition as well as treating appetite loss, constipation and indigestion.

Boneset contains vitamin C and the minerals calcium, magnesium and potassium. It also contains Para-Aminobenzoic Acid (PABA).

Historical Uses:	
Appetite Stimulant	Arthritis
Bacteria Infections	Bronchitis
Catarrh	Chills
Colds	Constipation
Fever Preventative	Flu
Immune System Support	Indigestion
Jaundice	Liver Problems
Malaria	Measles
Mumps	Muscular Rheumatism
Sore Throat	Tonic
Virus	Worms

Buchu

Plant Parts Used: Leaves

Buchu is native to South Africa, where it was used by native people as well as early colonists as a treatment for urinary tract infections. It has also been used for arthritis, cholera, kidney stones and muscle aches.

It is often combined with Cranberry to treat urinary tract infections.

Buchu is available in several over-the-counter diuretics for women who suffer from water retention before their periods. These medications are promoted as being useful to treat the bloating caused by premenstrual syndrome (PMS).

Historical Uses:	
Arthritis	Bed Wetting
Cystitis	Gallstones
Kidney Problems	Nephritis
Prostate Problems	Rheumatism
Urinary Tract Infections	

Buckthorn

Plant Parts Used: Bark & Berries

Buckthorn is a very potent laxative which was widely used in Europe during the 13th century. In more recent times it has been used for other purposes such as: arthritis, gout, hemorrhoids, jaundice and to promote menstruation.

When taken hot it induces sweating which will reduce a fever. When used as an ointment, the herb will reduce itching. If the leaves are bruised and applied to a wound it will stop small amounts of bleeding.

Historical Uses:	
Arthritis	Bowel Function
Constipation	External Warts
Fever	Gallstones
Gout	Hemorrhoids
Jaundice	Lead Poisoning
Liver Problems	Menstruation
Parasites	Rheumatism
Skin Diseases	Skin Irritation
Stops Bleeding	Worms

Burdock

Plant Parts Used: Root, Leaves and Seeds

Burdock Root is one of the best blood purifiers to clear circulatory and lymphatic congestion. As it assists in alleviating excess body fluids, toxins are more easily purged from the body.

Other uses for burdock root: aids in reducing swelling around joints, expels surplus calcium deposits and cleanses the blood of harmful acids. It has also been used to treat acne, dandruff, eczema, gonorrhea, gout, psoriasis, ringworm, skin infections, syphilis, and difficulties linked to childbirth.

Burdock contains vitamins A, B Complex, C, E, P and minerals copper, iodine, silicon, sulfur and zinc; as well as Para-Aminobenzoic Acid (PABA).

Historical Uses:	
Acne	Allergies
Arthritis	Asthma
Blood Purifier	Boils
Bronchitis	Childbirth
Circulatory System Support	Dandruff
Eczema	Fever
Gout	Hay Fever
Infections	Joint Inflammation
Kidney Problems	Liver Problems
Lungs	Lymphatic System Support
Nervousness	Rheumatism
Sexually Transmitted Diseases	Skin Disorders
Wound Healing	

Butchers Broom

Plant Parts Used: Root

Butchers Broom has been used for hundreds of years to provide support to the circulatory system—and with circulatory system conditions being the number one killer in the United States—this herb could prove very beneficial for many Americans.

Butchers Broom strengthens blood vessel walls, making it ideal in cases of post-operative surgery to prevent thrombosis. It is also used to treat hemorrhoids, phlebitis and varicose veins.

It increases blood circulation to the brain which can aid in memory function. Additionally, it can help prevent heart problems by reducing cholesterol levels and helping prevent atherosclerosis—a disease where plaque builds up inside arteries.

Historical Uses:	
Atherosclerosis	Brain (Blood Circulation)
Cholesterol Reduction	Circulatory System Support
Hemorrhoids	Memory
Phlebitis	Varicose Veins

Capsicum

Plant Parts Used: Fruit

Capsicum also called cayenne has a warming effect and is often used to treat instances of cold hands and cold feet. As such it is an excellent circulatory product. It has also gained a good reputation as a painkiller and digestive aid. The main active ingredient is capsaicin—an oily phytochemical. Capsicum is important in that it increases the power of all other herbs that have been consumed or applied. Additionally, it has been used to relieve symptoms of a cold and sore throat, as well as pyorrhea (inflammation of the gums.)

Capsicum contains vitamin A, B Complex, C, G; and minerals calcium, iron, magnesium, phosphorus, potassium and sulfur.

Historical Uses:	
Arthritis	Bleeding
Blood Cleanser	Bronchitis
Burns	Circulatory System Support
Colds	Congestion
Diabetes	Equalizers Blood Pressure
Expels Gas	Expels Mucus
Eyes	Fatigue
Fever	Heart Function
Infections	Jaundice
Kidney Problems	Pyorrhea
Pancreas Support	Tumor Fighter
Rheumatism	Sore Throat
Stroke	Ulcers
Varicose Veins	Wound Healing

Caraway

Plant Parts Used: Seeds

Caraway seed is something that is often thought of to add to rye bread. Why is it added to rye bread and other foods? The reason: since ancient times it has been used to support the digestive tract and expel gas.

In modern times, researchers have discovered that two oils in caraway seed—carvol and carvene—soothe the smooth muscle of the digestive tract, and it is these oils that make caraway so effective. Caraway is not only used to support the digestive system, but it also has an antispasmodic action which is a useful treatment for women who experience menstrual cramps.

Caraway contains vitamin B Complex, and minerals calcium, cobalt, copper, iodine, iron, magnesium, silicon and zinc.

Historical Uses:	
Colds	Colic
Digestion	Gas
Menstrual Cramps	Settles an upset Stomach
Spasms	Toothache
Uterine Cramps	

Cascara Sagrada

Plant Parts Used: Dried, Aged Bark

16th century explorers who first visited Northern California had a huge problem—they were severely constipated. Local Native Americans provided them with an herbal tea to help solve the problem. The tea worked so well with the result that the Spaniards named the herb Cascara Sagrada or "sacred bark."

Today, Cascara Sagrada is well known for its quick acting laxative effect. It is often used for constipation in addition to helping purge toxins from the body. It promotes peristaltic action—the movement of waste matter through the colon, and stimulates secretions from the gall bladder, liver, pancreas and stomach. Cascara Sagrada is considered a "very gentle" laxative, and is non-habit forming. It is especially useful where hemorrhoids are present due to poor bowel movements.

Historical Uses:	
Catarrh	Colon Cleansing
Constipation	Cough
Croup	Digestion
Dyspepsia	Expels Worms
Gall Bladder	Gallstones
Hemorrhoids	High Blood Pressure
Indigestion	Insomnia
Intestines	Jaundice
Liver Problems	Spleen

Catnip

Plant Parts Used: Flowers and Leaves

A member of the mint family, Catnip has been used for thousands of years from Europe to China. One of its main uses is to sooth the digestive tract, but also to alleviate the effects of a cold. American Indians used it for infant colic; and as it has a mild tranquilizer action, it has also been used to promote restful sleep, as well as provide support for the nervous system.

As Catnip is a spasmodic, it is often used to relieve menstrual cramps.

Catnip also possesses antibiotic properties which make it useful for treating diarrhea and to reduce the effects of a fever.

Catnip contains vitamin A, B Complex, C and minerals magnesium, manganese, phosphorus, sodium and sulfur.

Historic Uses:	
Anemia	Chronic Bronchitis
Colds	Colic
Convulsions	Cough
Diarrhea	Digestion
Expels Worms	Fatigue
Fever	Flu
Gas	Hemorrhoids
Hiccups	Improves Circulation
Lung congestion	Menstrual Cramps
Morning Sickness	Muscle Cramps
Nerves	Nervous Headaches
Nicotine withdrawal	Pain
Restlessness	Spasms
Stress	Upset Stomach
Vomiting	

Celery

Plant Parts Used: Root and Seeds

We often think of celery as something to add to salads to chew on—but researchers have found quite a few benefits in celery seeds. These benefits include: providing relief from anxiety and insomnia—Celery contains natural chemicals which have a sedative effect, Chinese researchers have successfully used Celery with people who suffer from high blood pressure. Various studies have shown that Celery Seed can reduce blood sugar (glucose) levels, which is an important component of managing diabetes.

Celery contains a natural diuretic which can help with weight loss—especially if someone is obese as it will tend to eliminate water weight. However, it is important to bear in mind that any water weight lost will tend to return. The only real answer to sustained—and maintained weight loss is to change the diet into one that is low in saturated fat and high in fiber and complex carbohydrates, coupled with an appropriate exercise program.

Celery contains vitamins A, B Complex, C and minerals calcium, iron, magnesium, phosphorus, potassium, silicon, sodium and sulfur.

Historical Uses:	
Anxiety	Diabetes
Dropsy	Headaches
Holding Urine	Insomnia
Liver Problems	Nasal Catarrh
Nervous System Disorders	Neuralgia
Rheumatism	Water Retention
Weight Loss	

Chamomile

Plant Parts Used: Flower

Dried chamomile flowers were used in ancient Egypt, Greece and Rome to treat many disorders of the body including anxiety, stress and sleeping problems. This was achieved by its calming and sedative effect. In more recent times it has been used as a tea for relaxation and as a sleep aid.

Chamomile has an antispasmodic action which means in is highly beneficial for supporting the digestive system. Studies done on animals suggest that this herb could help prevent stomach ulcers and increase their healing rate.

Another use for its antispasmodic action is as an aid to relieve the effects of menstrual cramps. It also helps relieve arthritis pain by reducing inflammation in the joints. Children can benefit from Chamomile as it is a useful aid for colds, stomach problems, colitis, as a gargle and applied externally for skin inflammation and eczema.

Early American settlers used a Chamomile compress to prevent wounds becoming infected. Studies show that Chamomile Oil reduces the time it takes burns to heal, and other studies show that the herb can kill Candida Albicans yeast.

And finally, Chamomile supports the Immune System by stimulating macrophages and B-Lymphocytes—white blood cells whose purpose is to fight internal body infections.

Chamomile contains vitamin A and minerals calcium, iron, magnesium, manganese, potassium and zinc.

Historical Uses:	
Anxiety	Arthritis
Candida Yeast Infections	Colds
Colitis	Digestive System Support
Eczema	Immune System Support
Menstrual Cramps	Stomach Ulcers
Skin Inflammation	Throat Gargle
Wound Healing	

Chaparral

Plant Parts Used: Leaves and Stems

Chaparral has very strong antioxidant properties in addition to it being an antiseptic, pain killer and having anti-tumor actions.

In its antiseptic form, it is often used as a mouthwash to fight tooth decay, and pyorrhea—inflammation of the gums. One study shows that a Chaparral mouthwash reduced cavities by 75 percent.

As a tumor fighter the National Cancer Institute has received numerous testimonials from different individuals claiming that it cured their cancers. In fact several studies have shown that in fact it does shrink cancer tumors.

Chaparral contains minerals aluminum, barium, chlorine, potassium, sodium, sulfur and tin. It is also an excellent source of protein.

Historical Uses:	
Aches	Arthritis
Bad Breath	Blood Cleanser
Cancer Fighter	Gum Disease
Mouthwash	Pain Killer
Tumor Fighter	

Chickweed

Plant Parts Used: Whole Herb

Chickweed is used to strengthen the colon and stomach as well as helping to dissolve plaque and fatty deposits. Because of its mucilage content, Chickweed has healing properties for stomach ulcers and inflammation in the colon.

It can also be used as a poultice for burns, boils and skin conditions, and has often been referred to as efficient anti-cancer agent.

Chickweed contains vitamin B Complex, C, D and minerals calcium, copper, iron, magnesium, phosphorus and zinc.

Historical Uses:	
Anti-Cancer Properties	Arteriosclerosis
Blood Cleanser	Boils
Burns	Constipation
Intestinal Health	Skin Conditions
Stomach Ulcers	

Cloves

Plant Parts Used: Seeds, dried powdered flower buds

Cloves are a good natural parasite cleansing herb which can be obtained as a liquid, powder or in a capsule.

As a liquid it is often rubbed on to the gums to relieve toothache, it is also an excellent remedy for bad breath.

It is also a good herb to use to support the digestive system due to its ability to help relax the smooth muscle lining the digestive tract.

Cloves are one of the most potent germicidal agents available in herbal form.

Cloves contain vitamin A, B Complex, C and minerals calcium, magnesium, phosphorus, potassium and sodium.

Historical Uses:	
Bad Breath	Digestive System Support
Expel Parasites	Gum Problems
Toothache	

Coltsfoot

Plant Parts Used: Leaves and Flowers

Coltsfoot is best known as a cough suppressant and to support the respiratory system. This herb has a high mucilage and saponin content which acts as a disinfectant and anti-inflammatory agent for respiratory problems.

The flowers have expectorant properties which mean they are very soothing to mucus membranes and are especially beneficial for chest and lung conditions.

Coltsfoot contains vitamin A, B6 (Pyridoxine), B12 (Cyanocobalamin), C, P and minerals calcium, copper, iron, manganese and potassium.

Historical Uses:	
Bronchitis	Catarrh
Chest Conditions	Colds
Cough	Lung Inflammation
Mucus	Pneumonia
Respiratory Problems	

Comfrey

Plant Parts Used: Leaves and Root

Comfrey contains a chemical called Allantoin which helps with the growth of new cells. This chemical is the reason why Comfrey is well known as a wound healer and to knit broken bones together, Comfrey has been used for centuries for these two purposes.

As Comfrey secretes its natural hormone to the pituitary gland, it helps to strengthen the structural system.

Comfrey also supports the digestive system by helping the secretion of pepsin and it is a general aid for the respiratory system. In fact, Comfrey is a general aid and tonic for the whole body.

Historical Uses:	
Bleeding	Broken Bones
Burns	Digestive System Disorders
Fractures	Respiratory System Problems
Sores	Stomach Problems
Structural System Support	Tonic
Ulcers (Internal & External)	Wound Healing

Cranberry

Plant Parts Used: Juice from the berries

Cranberry main purpose is to treat bacterial infections in the bladder. It is often combined with buchu herb.

When used together, these two herbs have anti-inflammatory, diuretic and antiseptic properties. Scientific studies show that cranberry makes the urinary tract inhospitable to bacteria, lessening the risk of urinary tract infections. Buchu acts as a diuretic and improves digestion. This product works best in acidic urine conditions.

Cranberry is rich in vitamin C

Historical Uses:	
Incontinence	Scurvy
Urinary Tract Infections	

Damiana

Plant Parts Used: Leaves

Damiana is one of the most popular herbal products to restore normal sexual function in males by increasing sperm count, and for strengthening the egg in females. In addition, it helps to balance female hormones. It is helpful in increasing sexual strength in those who have a weak libido.

Historical Uses:	
Balances Female Hormones	Exhaustion
Female Problems	Frigidity
Hot Flashes	Lack of Libido
Male Problems	Parkinson's Disease
Prostate Support	Sexual Energy

Dandelion

Plant Parts Used: Leaves and Root

Dandelion is very often thought of as a weed in the garden—to be destroyed if possible. However, it has been used for centuries to stimulate the liver to detoxify poisons. It is important for promoting good circulatory system function and strengthening weak arteries.

Dandelion has a diuretic action which can be helpful in cases of premenstrual syndrome, and it can be helpful in a weight loss program for those who carry excess water. Although as mentioned elsewhere in this book, water will often return. Diuretics are often prescribed for high blood pressure therefore Dandelion may have a role to play here as well.

One study determined that Dandelion inhibits the growth of a fungus that is implicated in the growth of Candida Albicans yeast infections.

In Germany physicians often prescribe Dandelion to increase the flow of bile and thus reduce the risk of gallstones.

Dandelion contains vitamin A, B Complex, C, E and minerals calcium, cobalt, copper, iron, nickel, potassium, sodium, tin and zinc.

Historical Uses:	
Candida Yeast Infections	Circulatory System Support
Cramps	Detoxify Poisons
Gallstones	High Blood Pressure
Liver Stimulant	Premenstrual Syndrome
Purifies the Blood	Weak Arteries
Weight Loss	

Dong Quai

Plant Parts Used: Root

Dong Quai – a member of the celery family - is one of the oldest known herbs, having been used in China, Japan and Korea for over 1,000 years. It is primarily known as a women's product, to relieve menopausal symptoms such as: hot flashes, menstrual disorders such as cramps, irregular menstrual cycles, infrequent periods, premenstrual syndrome (PMS), and menopausal symptoms.

It is suggested that Dong Quai contains compounds that may help reduce pain, dilate blood vessels, and stimulate and relax uterine muscles.

In traditional Chinese medicine (TCM), different parts of the dong quai root are used for different actions in the body: the root head is used as an anticoagulant, the main part of the root is used as a tonic, and the tail-end of the root is used to remove blood stagnation. Because it is a balancer of the female hormonal system, it is often called "female's ginseng."

Dong Quai contains vitamin A, B12 (Cyanocobalamin) and E.

Historical Uses:	
Abdominal Aches	Blood Clots
Circulatory System Support	Cramps
Female Reproductive Glands	Hot Flashes
High Blood Pressure	Internal Bleeding
Menopause	Metabolism
Migraine Headaches	Nervous System Support
Nourishes the Brain	Regulates Menstruation
Tonic	

Echinacea

Plant Parts Used: Root

There are various strains of Echinacea. It is used to support the immune system and is involved in the production of white blood cells, which assists the body in fight infection. Echinacea purges toxins from the blood and enhances lymphatic drainage.

Echinacea contains polysaccharides that stimulate the production of phagocytes (cells that engulf and consume foreign matter) and activate T -lymphocytes, macrophages and natural killer cells. Taken at the earliest sign of a cold or infection, echinacea may help cut recovery time considerably.

Echinacea contains vitamin A, C, E and minerals copper, iodine, iron, potassium and sulfur.

Historical Uses:	
Arthritis	Bites
Cancer	Candida Yeast Infections
Colds	Eczema
Flu	Infections
Lymph Glands	Purifies the Blood
Radiation Therapy	Stings
Tumors	Wound Healing

Elderflower

Plant Parts Used: Berries and Flowers

One of the oldest known herbs. It works in the respiratory and immune body systems, and is usually used to counter the effects of colds, flu, congestion, sore throat and inflammation.

In addition, it also rids the cells of toxic waste, and it also acts to reduce fever and is a support for the circulatory system by increasing blood circulation.

Elderflower contains alkaloids which have a mild sedative action as well as being a pain reliever, expectorant and having anti-inflammatory properties as well.

It is suitable for babies, children, adults and the elderly.

Elderflower contains vitamin A and C as well as bioflavonoids.

Historical Uses:	
Asthma	Bronchitis
Colds	Congested Sinuses
Digestive System Disorders	Fever
Flu	Nervous Conditions
Pneumonia	Swollen Joints

Elecampane

Plant Parts Used: Root

Used for over 1,000 years, Elecampane is probably best known for expelling intestinal parasites and worms. But that is not all; it is also effective as a respiratory system support—especially for the elimination of catarrh. As it is one of the richest natural sources of insulin it is highly beneficial for the pancreas.

Elecampane contains minerals calcium, potassium and sodium.

Historical Uses:	
Asthma	Bronchitis
Catarrh	Digestive System Support
Expels Parasites	Expels Phlegm
Expels Worms	

Eucalyptus

Plant Parts Used: Leaf Oil

Have you ever used Listerine mouthwash or Vicks VapaRub, if so then you have come into contact with Eucalyptus? Eucalyptus Oil is very potent and is therefore excellent for loosening phlegm in the chest, making it easier for it to be expelled. It is also used to treat cases of pyorrhea—inflammation of the gums.

Eucalyptus provides an anti-bacterial action against infections in minor cuts and wounds. Studies in Russia have determined that Eucalyptus kills the influenza virus.

Historical Uses:	
Antiseptic	Burns
Catarrh	Colds
Expels Worms	External Ulcers
Fever	Flu
Infections	Mouthwash
Pyorrhea	Sore Throat
Wound Healing	

Fennel

Plant Parts Used: Fruits (Seeds). Bulbs and Stalks are used in cooking

Fennel Seed has several uses including: supporting the digestive system where—like most aromatic herbs—it has the ability to relax the smooth muscle lining the digestive tract; it also assists in expelling gas and helps with intestinal problems. Fennel also supports the nervous systems, alleviates the effects of colic, and it also has diuretic properties.

Studies show that Fennel has mild estrogenic effects similar to the female sex hormone estrogen.

Fennel contains the minerals potassium, sodium and sulfur.

Historical Uses:	
Bronchitis	Colic
Congestion	Cough
Digestive System Support	Expels Gas
Female Problems	Intestinal System Disorders
Nervous System Support	

Fenugreek

Plant Parts Used: Seeds

Fenugreek comprises various components including saponins, alkaloids and fiber. It is a respiratory system herb which assists in expelling mucous, phlegm and infections from the lungs, and toxic waste through the lymphatic system. In addition, Fenugreek is able to dissolve a hardened build-up of mucous which can then be eliminated.

Fenugreek has a mild anti-inflammatory action which makes it especially useful in treating arthritis and wounds. In addition, Fenugreek contains mucilage which can help relief a sore throat.

As Fenugreek contains lecithin and other fat dissolving compounds, it has the ability to emulsify cholesterol and other fat deposits that build up in the arteries which if left untreated can ultimately lead to heart disease or a stroke.

Fenugreek contains vitamin A, B1 (Thiamine), B2 (Riboflavin), B3 (Niacin) and D, as well as having significant quantities of various minerals. It also contains lecithin, choline and has a significant protein content. It also contains an oil that is very similar to cod liver oil.

Historical Uses:	
Arthritis	Catarrh
Cholesterol Reduction	Colds
Cough	Fatty Deposits
Inflammation	Lung Infections
Phlegm	Respiratory System Support
Sore Throat	Toxic Waste Removal
Wound Healing	

Garcinia Cambogia

Plant Parts Used: Fruit

Garcinia Cambogia is a tropical fruit which contains HCA (hydroxy-citric acid), which stimulates the body to burn carbohydrates as energy rather than storing them as fat. HCA acts as an appetite suppressant which reduces the intake of food, thus reducing fat and cholesterol formation.

Historical Uses:	
Appetite Suppressant	Carbohydrate Reduction
Fat Burning	Weight Loss

Garlic

Plant Parts Used: Bulb

This popular herb offers a boost to the immune system with its antibacterial, antifungal and antiviral properties. It is excellent for purging candida yeast and parasites from the body.

Garlic has so many uses from using it in cooking to it being an excellent product for heart health. Other recognized health benefits of garlic include, acting as an antibiotic and having anti-cholesterol and anti-hypertensive properties.

It is also an antioxidant which protects the body against the effects of free radical damage. Its high sulfur content assists in cell purification.

Allicin is the principle biological active compound which gives garlic its odor. Be warned. Many so called "odorless" garlic products have the active compound removed which makes it rather worthless. It can be obtained as a garlic bulb, in a capsule or in tablet form.

- For respiratory conditions use with mullein or lobelia
- For bacterial infection use with golden seal, echinacea, Pau d'Arco
- As a decongestant / expectorant use with lobelia
- For parasites use with pumpkin seeds and black walnut
- For swollen lymph nodes use with lobelia and mullein
- For viral infections use with colloidal silver
- For yeast infections use with Pau d'Arco

Historical Uses:	
Anti-bacterial	Anti-biotic - natural penicillin
Anti-Viral	Arteriosclerosis
Arthritis	Asthma
Athletes Foot	Blood poisoning
High Blood Pressure	Parasites

Gentian

Plant Parts Used: Root

Gentian Root helps in the breakdown of fats and proteins and assists in the body's assimilation of iron and vitamin B12. As it has a cooling effect on body tissue, this helps reduce infections and inflammation. Gentian Root also promotes digestive secretions.

Gentian also supports the circulatory system and is an excellent stomach tonic. It also contains natural sugar which is useful for pancreas and spleen support.

One Chinese study showed that Gentian has excellent anti-inflammatory properties and has been prescribed successfully for arthritic conditions.

Historical Uses:	
Arthritis	Blood Strengthener
Circulatory System Support	Digestive System Support
Fever	Infections
Inflamed Joints	Pancreas Support
Spleen Support	Stomach Support

Ginger

Plant Parts Used: Root

Ginger Root is an excellent cleansing agent for the colon, skin and kidneys. Many people take it as a natural alternative for motion and morning sickness.

Ginger also supports the digestive system, and is an excellent herb for abdominal cramping and indigestion. Due to its anti-spasmodic action, it may help ease menstrual cramps.

As Ginger also contains anti-inflammatory compounds, it has been successfully used to treat arthritis. Ginger also helps lower cholesterol as well as high blood pressure and reduces the risk of blood clots forming which could trigger a heart attack or stroke.

Ginger has proved successful for expelling phlegm and as such, is used to treat asthma, bronchitis, colds, flu and congestion of the respiratory system.

It also has a microbial action. In studies Ginger has shown to be effective in eradicating bacteria and parasites including flukes, roundworms and tapeworms.

When applied topically, Ginger helps reduce heat in inflamed joints. Ginger supports the circulatory system and by detoxifying the blood it reduces the debilitating effects of arthritis and rheumatism.

Ginger contains vitamin A, B Complex, C and minerals calcium, iron, manganese, phosphorus, potassium and sodium.

Historical Uses:	
Arthritis	Asthma
Bacteria Infections	Bronchitis
Colds	Cough
Diarrhea	Digestive System Support
Fever	Flatulence
Flu	Indigestion
Loss of Appetite	Morning Sickness
Motion Sickness	Parasites
Respiratory System Support	Rheumatism
Worms	

Ginkgo Biloba

Plant Parts Used: Leaves

Ginkgo Biloba—an antioxidant herb—promotes increased circulation. It also dilates blood vessels and bronchioles to improve circulation and oxygenation of cells. It also has scientifically proven nervous system benefits in addition to improving memory function by increasing blood flow to the brain.

Those individuals who suffer from tinnitus "ringing in the ears" have had beneficial results due to Ginkgo's ability to increase blood flow to the nerves in the inner ear.

Ginkgo is also good for the heart as it increases blood flow to the heart muscle which has the effect of reducing the risk of blood clots forming which can trigger a heart attack.

The eyes also benefit too! Ginkgo increases blood flow to the retina in the eye which can help reduce the risk of macular degeneration—one of the leading causes of blindness in adults, especially as they age.

In one study men who had problems gaining and maintaining an erection found that by taking Ginkgo they were able to achieve a normal sustained erection. Impotence is often caused by narrowing of the arteries that supply blood to the penis.

Historical Uses:	
Circulatory System Support	Dizziness
Erectile Dysfunction	Eyes
Heart Support	Impotence
Memory	Stroke
Tinnitus	Varicose Veins
Vertigo	

Ginseng

Plant Parts Used: Root

There is not just one Ginseng but three, although all three are often referred to as "Ginseng". The three varieties are: Korean (Panax Ginseng), American Ginseng and Siberian Ginseng (Eleutherococcus). Technically Siberian Ginseng is not a true Ginseng, however, it contains similar active compounds to the other two and achieves similar effects, and so all three are grouped together as Ginseng.

The active chemicals in Ginseng are called ginsenosides and it is these that provide the majority of benefits.

One of the benefits of Ginseng is its therapeutic ability to protect the body against the effects of stress, radiation and chemical toxins.

Ginseng also supports the immune system to stimulate white blood cells (macrophages and natural killer cells) to go and do battle against disease causing micro-organisms. Ginseng also stimulates the body to produce interferon—its own natural chemical to fight against bacterial and viral attacks.

Ginseng helps reduce blood sugar levels which can make it useful as part of a diabetic management program. It is also a good liver protector, helping protect it from the effects of alcohol, drugs and other toxic substances. Ginseng can help protect cells against the effects of radiation due to cancer radiation therapy.

Ginseng also has Aphrodisiac properties, and some studies show that those who take the herb are more sexually active than those who don't take it.

Historical Uses:	
Aphrodisiac	Appetite Stimulant
Cancer	Chemical Toxins
Diabetes	Effects of Radiation
Energy	Heart Protector
Immune System Support	Lowers Cholesterol
Stress	

Golden Seal

Plant Parts Used: Rhizome and Root

Golden Seal has two active alkaloids—berberine and hydrastine. Berberine is also the active ingredient in Barberry (which is featured earlier in this book). Therefore, Barberry and Goldenseal are used for similar things—however Barberry is a lot cheaper than Goldenseal.

Golden Seal has astringent properties which produces a vasoconstricting effect—or tightening of blood vessels. It is the alkaloid hydrastine mentioned above which gives Goldenseal its astringent properties. This alkaloid also stimulates the autonomic nervous system.

Golden Seal's astringent qualities are useful in the toning of mucus membranes. This then helps with ear, eye, nose and throat problems. Other problems which can be addressed by utilizing Golden Seal's astringent properties include: intestinal and stomach disorders as well as prostate gland and vaginal problems

Golden Seal facilitates the secretion of digestive enzymes as well as fluids—especially bile which assists in the regulation of liver and spleen function.

In studies Golden Seal has been show to assist with the healing of damaged skin tissue from the effects of acne, eczema, rashes, smallpox and other sores or wounds. Golden Seal has been used successfully to treat outbreaks of herpes in the genital area (genital herpes).

Historical Uses:	
Acne	Digestive System Support
Ear Problems	Eczema
Eye Problems	Genital Herpes
Intestinal System Disorders	Liver Function
Nervous System Problems	Nose Problems
Prostate Problems	Rashes
Smallpox	Spleen Function
Stomach Problems	Throat Problems
Vaginal Problems	Wound Healing

Gotu Kola

Plant Parts Used: Leaves

Gotu Kola originates from Sri Lanka. It is used extensively in Ayurvedic medicine where its prime purpose is to support the nervous system and especially the brain. It is therefore often referred to as "food for the brain". It is a nervous system tonic where it generates energy within the cells of the brain, and as a result, it escalates physical and mental power as well as stimulating the pituitary gland.

Gotu Kola's primary use for centuries was to treat serious skin conditions such as bruises, elephantitis and leprosy (which is now called Hansen's disease), psoriasis and syphilitic ulcers.

A study published in the British journal Nature supported the use of Gotu Kola for the treatment of leprosy. The bacteria that causes leprosy has a waxy coating which protects them from white blood cells in the immune system designed to destroy them. Gotu Kola contains a chemical (asiaticoside) which destroy this wax coating which enables the bacteria to be destroyed.

A cream containing Gotu Kola applied to painful scaly psoriasis welts can bring relief. Various studies have shown that Gotu Kola improves circulation in the lower limbs. Further studies are underway to determine if Gotu Kola would be suitable for treating varicose veins.

Gotu Kola contains vitamin B3 (Niacin), K, and minerals calcium, magnesium, manganese, silicon and sodium.

Historical Uses:	
Ayurvedic Medicine	Blood Circulation
Brain	Bruises
Circulatory System	Elephantitis
Epilepsy	Hansen's Disease
Leprosy	Memory Loss
Nervous System Problems	Nervous System Support
Pituitary Gland	Schizophrenia,
Varicose Veins	

Gymnema Sylvestre

Plant Parts Used: Leaf

Gymnema Sylvestre is a climbing plant which is native to Australia, parts of Africa and central and southern India, and is used in Ayurvedic medicine. It is primarily used for weight management to control appetite and cravings, but has also been used to treat constipation and is one of the most effective complementary therapies for managing type 1 and type 11 diabetes.

In cases of type 1 and type 11 diabetes it assists in the regulation of elevated or fluctuating blood sugar levels. Gymnema assists the pancreas in the production of insulin by increasing the regeneration of insulin-producing beta cells to control glucose levels.

Gymnema Sylvestre has also been shown to reduce blood cholesterol and triglyceride levels without noticeable side effects. Additionally, Ayurvedic doctors use Gymnema to treat cases of allergies, anemia, coughs, obesity, osteoporosis and urinary system disorders,

Historical Uses:	
Allergies	Anemia
Appetite Suppressant	Ayurvedic Medicine
Blood Sugar Levels	Constipation
Cough	Diabetes
Obesity	Osteoporosis
Reduces Cholesterol	Sugar Cravings
Triglyceride Levels	Urinary System Disorders
Weight Management	

Hawthorn

Plant Parts Used: Flowers, Leaves, Fruits

The seventeenth-century English herbalist Nicolas Culpeper described Hawthorn as "a singular remedy for the stone (kidney stones), and no less effective for dropsy (congestive heart failure)".

Hawthorn is known as the heart herb. It improves circulation and heart strength. In studies, hawthorn recipients also reported fewer overall symptoms, less fatigue and less shortness of breath.

In fact it supports the heart in various ways. It can open the coronary arteries thus improving blood supply to the heart. It can increase the heart's pumping force, and it may help limit the amount of cholesterol deposited on arterial walls.

However, Hawthorn is not a quick fix for the heart. It takes time for benefits to accumulate—but the benefits are worth it in the long run.

Hawthorn is often taken along with ginkgo biloba to improve circulation especially to the heart.

Hawthorn contains vitamin B Complex, C, and minerals aluminum, beryllium, iron, nickel sulfur, tin and zinc.

Historical Uses:	
Angina	Arteriosclerosis
Cholesterol Reduction	Congestive Heart Failure
Enlarged Heart	Hardening of the Arteries
Heart Palpitations	High Blood Pressure
Kidney Problems	

Hibiscus

Plant Parts Used: Flower

Hibiscus is used for a multitude of medical conditions including: circulatory system disorders, as a diuretic to increase urine flow, in the respiratory system for expelling phlegm, for nervous system disorders, stomach irritation, colds and flu, heart conditions and loss of appetite. Some researchers speculate that Hibiscus could contain alkaloids that have an antibiotic action to kill bacteria and worms, and additional alkaloids to treat cases of high blood pressure.

Historical Uses:	
Bacteria Infections	Circulatory System Disorders
Colds	Diuretic
Flu	Heart Health
Loss of Appetite	Nervous System Disorders
Urinary System Disorders	Worms

Hops

Plant Parts Used: Flower

Hops have three primary medicinal functions: as a sedative, digestive aid and for women health. Of the three, it is best known for its sedative qualities on the nervous system, and for inducing sleep in cases of insomnia.

According to French researchers, Hops has antispasmodic properties which improves digestion by relaxes the muscle lining of the digestive tract.

German researchers state that Hops contains alkaloids similar to the female sex hormone estrogen which promotes menstruation.

Hops contain vitamin B Complex and minerals chlorine, copper, fluorine, iodine, iron, lead, magnesium, manganese, sodium and zinc.

Historical Uses:	
Anxiety	Digestive System Support
Hyperactivity	Insomnia
Menstruation	Nervous System Support
Sleep	

Horehound

Plant Parts Used: Leaves and Flower Tops

Horehound has been used for over 2000 years as an herbal expectorant and cough remedy. Horehound contains an alkaloid (marrubiin) which loosens phlegm. Horehound also has the ability to stimulate bile secretions and is also used for wound healing.

Horehound acts as a tonic to the respiratory system as well as the stomach. It has also been used successfully when applied topically for such skin conditions as the herpes simplex virus, eczema and shingles.

Horehound contains vitamin A, B Complex, C, E, F and minerals iron, potassium and sulfur.

Historical Uses:	
Bronchitis	Cold
Cough	Eczema applied topically
Expectorant for Phlegm	Herpes Simplex Virus applied topically
Shingles applied topically	Wound Healing

Horsetail

Plant Parts Used: Stems

This herb has diuretic properties and can help with some kidney conditions. It is particularly effective for healing when blood is present in the urine. Horsetail also has astringent properties and as such, is used for bed-wetting in children and incontinence in Adults.

Horsetail is rich in silica, which helps to soothe and strengthen connective tissue. Silica is required for bone and cartilage formation, as well as assisting the body in absorbing and utilizing calcium. Calcium is needed for repairing fractures and treating bone diseases, including rickets and osteoporosis. Horsetail is used to strengthen bones, teeth, nails and hair. The improved cartilage helps to lessen inflammation and combat joint pain, arthritis, gout, muscle cramps, hemorrhoids, spasms and rheumatism.

The silica content in Horsetail also promotes the growth of collagen—a protein found in connective tissue, Collagen assists in improving skin health and tone.

Horsetail contains vitamin B5 (Pantothenic Acid), E and minerals cobalt, copper, iodine, iron, manganese, selenium, silica, sodium, as well as Para-Aminobenzoic Acid (PABA).

Historical Uses;	
Bed Wetting	Brittle Nails
Circulatory System Disorders	Hair Condition (split ends)
Incontinence	Kidney Problems
Skin Conditions	Strengthen Bones
Strengthen Teeth	Urinary System Disorders
Urinary Tract Infections	

Hydrangea

Plant Parts Used: Leaves and Root

Hydrangea is best known as a treatment for kidney and bladder stones. Kidney stones are made of mineral and acid salts which form into hard deposits inside the kidneys. Many things can cause kidney stones to form, but one of the most common causes is not drinking enough fluids during the day—ideally filtered water.

Most often kidney stones form when the urine becomes concentrated and this allows minerals to crystalize and clump together. Hydrangea helps stop these deposits from forming—which cause severe pain when they pass from the kidneys through the ureters to the bladder.

Recent studies show that Hydrangea can reduce inflammation of the prostate gland and improve prostate health. Adding Horsetail can increase the effectiveness of the treatment.

Herbalists recommend Hydrangea for many conditions of the urinary system including: cystitis, benign prostatic hyperplasia (BPH), dysuria, edema, incontinence, inflammation and tumor formation.

Hydrangea contains minerals calcium, chromium, iron, magnesium, phosphorus, potassium, sodium and sulfur.

Historical Uses:	
Benign Prostatic Hyperplasia (BPH)	Edema
Incontinence	Kidney Stones
Prostate Health	Tumors
Urinary Tract Infections	

Hyssop

Plant Parts Used: Leaves and Flowers

You can find Hyssop mentioned several times in the Bible. For example in the Book of Leviticus 14:1-7 *"Thus the priest shall look, and if the infection of leprosy has been healed in the leper, then the priest shall give orders to take two live clean birds and cedar wood and a scarlet string and hyssop for the one who is to be cleansed."*

There is more to "cleaning" than mentioned in the Bible. In fact Hyssop is often used to induce sweating to reduce fevers; and leaves can be applied to wounds to help reduce infections and assist in the healing process.

Hyssop has been used successfully as a gargle to treat nose and throat infections, and used as an infusion for a cough, where phlegm and congestion are involved, which develops from having a cold. Camphor-like compounds in Hyssop help to expectorate phlegm. It is also an aid for poor digestion as well as to treat breast and lung problems. It has also been used to expel mucus in the intestines.

Used as an infusion in a compress Hyssop restricts the growth of the Herpes Simplex virus which causes cold sores, as well as the Genital Herpes virus.

Historical Uses:	
Breast Problems	Cold Sores
Colds	Cough
Digestive System Disorders	Fever
Genital Herpes	Herpes Simplex Virus
Lung Problems	Nose Infections
Throat Infections	

Juniper

Plant Parts used: Berries

Juniper is used for several conditions in herbal healing. In the urinary system, because Juniper contains a chemical terpinene-4-0l which has diuretic properties, it is often used where uric acid is being retained in addition to excess water retention; it is also used to treat cases of high blood pressure.

Diuretics assist in relieving the bloated feeling caused by premenstrual fluid retention. Females concerned with premenstrual syndrome may obtain benefits by trying Juniper during the stressful days prior to their monthly periods.

Juniper has been found to be especially useful for treating prostate and urinary tract infections in men who suffer from benign prostatic hypertrophy (BPH). It is also a useful herb for treating cases of bacteria and yeast infections.

A liquid extract can be made from Juniper Berries and used as a gargle for mouth and throat infections.

Juniper also has anti-inflammatory properties which makes it a useful herb for arthritic conditions.

Because of its high chromium content, Juniper has also been used to treat blood sugar imbalances.

Juniper contains vitamin C, and minerals aluminum, cobalt, copper, chromium, sulfur and tin.

Historical Uses:	
Arthritis	Bacterial Infections
Blood Sugar Imbalance	Mouth Infections
Premenstrual Syndrome	Throat Infections
Urinary System Support	Urinary Tract Infections
Yeast Infections	

Kava Kava

Plant Parts Used: Root

Kava Kava has been used for hundreds of years in the Pacific Islands as a ceremonial drink. Reports suggest that the effect is similar to having an alcoholic drink.

The roots are either chewed or ground into a pulp and then added to cold water. When ground into a pulp, the thick brew is then offered to guests on social occasions.

As well as being used on ceremonial occasions, Kava is best known for its relaxing effect. Kava enhances mood and projects a feeling of well-being. Various studies have determined that Kava is a useful herb for the treatment of anxiety, insomnia and other nervous system disorders as it offers a natural sedative effect, which does not affect alertness unlike some medications.

However, there has been some concern in recent years that Kava could cause liver damage. This was based on some misguided studies which were done in Germany. And as a result without any further research, mainland Europe and the United Kingdom, as well as Canada have misguidedly banned the sale of Kava even though it has been used safely for hundreds of years in the Pacific Islands.

Fortunately, the FDA in the United States took a more pragmatic approach, and conduced their own studies, which showed that if the safe part of the herb is used—which is the root and not the stems or leaves—then Kava can be used safely. The FDA has even gone as far as to recommend safe dosage amounts of approximately 290 milligrams per day. This is interesting as it sets Kava apart from other herbal products which are recommended for insomnia and other anxiety disorders which carry no dosage recommendations at all.

However, Kava Kava should not be taken for more than six months at a time unless advised otherwise by a qualified practitioner.

Historical Uses:	
Anxiety	Insomnia
Nervous System Disorders	

Kelp

Plant Parts Used: The Whole Plant

Kelp is a sea vegetable which is harvested at low tide. It is an excellent source of iodine and in 1750 a British physician introduced a cure for goiter—a thyroid enlargement caused by thyroid deficiency—by mixing vegetable oil with charred kelp. In fact no one knew how his concoction worked until 1812 when scientists realized there was iodine in the kelp plant and that goiters were caused by iodine deficiency.

In fact Kelp provides good support for the glandular system, as it assists with control of the thyroid gland and helps regulate the metabolism which is involved with food digestion.

Kelp contains sodium alginate which is beneficial for health issues associated with heavy metal toxicity, radiation and heart disease.

In addition to the above, kelp also has many uses including: anemia, arthritis, asthma, candida yeast infections, coughs, diabetes, prostate and ovarian problems, fatigue, fungal infections, high blood pressure, ulcers and skin conditions such as eczema and psoriasis.

Kelp is a rich source of nutrients including: almost every mineral and trace mineral needed by the body,;vitamin A, B Complex, C, D, E, G, K, S; essential fatty acids, protein, amino acids and carbohydrates.

Historical Uses:	
Anemia	Arthritis
Asthma	Blood Cleanser
Candida Yeast Infections	Cough
Diabetes	Digestive System Support
Eczema	Energy
Fatigue	Fungal Infections
Glandular System Support	Goiter
Heart Disease	Heavy Metal Toxicity
High Blood Pressure	Obesity
Ovarian problems	Prostate Problems
Psoriasis	Radiation
Thyroid Problems	Ulcers

Kudzu

Plant Parts Used: Root

Historically Asian-Healers have used Kudzu to treat colds, flu, high blood pressure, allergies and many other ailments.

More recently, Chinese-Healers have used Kudzu to treat people who have an alcohol dependency. It has also been used with St John's Wort to treat the depressive effects of alcohol withdrawal. Kudzu is available in capsules, tablets, and dried root.

Historical Uses:	
Alcohol Withdrawal	Allergies
Colds	Flu
High Blood Pressure	

Lavender

Plant Parts Used: Stems, Flowers

Lavender can be used in different ways to treat anxiety, tension, headaches and insomnia. It is usually steeped in hot water so that the steam can be inhaled. Other options are to make it into a tea or it can be used as an essential oil and massaged into the skin. This will help manage stress and improve mood, concentration and reduce anxiety. Lavender has the ability to relax the nervous system and improve sleep patterns.

Historical Uses:	
Anxiety	Headaches
Insomnia	Nervous System Support
Relaxing	Stress

Lemon Balm

Plant Parts Used: Leaves

Lemon Balm is a member of the mint family and the leaves have a mild lemon aroma. Lemon Balm has several uses including: supporting the digestive system—colic, bloating, intestinal gas, stomach upset, and vomiting.

Lemon Balm is also used to support the nervous system in cases of anxiety, insomnia and restlessness; it is also used for Alzheimer's disease, in cases involving attention deficit-hyperactivity disorder (ADHD), and for Graves' Disease which is an autoimmune disorder involving the thyroid gland.

Other uses include: reducing high blood pressure, rapid heartbeat due to nervousness, swollen airways, sores as well as tumors. Individuals have also applied Lemon Balm to their skin to treat cases of cold sores linked to the Herpes Simplex Virus.

Historical Uses:	
Anxiety	Bloating
Cold Sores	Colic
Digestive System Disorders	Graves' Disease
Herpes Simplex Virus	Insomnia
Intestinal Gas	Nervous System Support
Restlessness	Stomach Upset
Thyroid Problems	Vomiting

Licorice

Plant Parts Used: Root

Licorice has long been recognized for the natural sweetness of its deep-sinking roots (Its Greek name of "sweet root" is very apt, as it is 50 times sweeter than sugar). Next to ginseng, licorice is the most popular herb used in Chinese formulas. It helps support the adrenal glands during periods of stress. Licorice is also a source of the female sex hormone estrogen.

Licorice contains glycosides which have the ability to purge excess fluid from the body—but especially the lungs and throat. It is an excellent herb when recovering from illness as it supplies energy to the body.

It helps alleviate inflammation in the intestinal tract and will act as a mild laxative. It can also relieve ulcer conditions and reduce instances of stress.

Licorice stimulates cell production of the body's own natural antiviral compound interferon which makes it especially useful in cases of cold sores caused by the Herpes Simplex virus as well as sores associated with Genital Herpes. Sprinkling dried Licorice Root powder on to clean sores may help to speed up healing.

Licorice contains vitamin B Complex, Biotin, B3 (Niacin), B5 (Pantothenic Acid), E, and minerals: chromium, iodine, manganese and zinc. It is also a source of lecithin.

Historical Uses:	
Adrenal Gland Support	Cold Sores
Energy	Genital Herpes
Herpes Simplex Virus	Inflammation
Intestinal System Disorders	Laxative Action
Stress	

Lobelia

Plant Parts Used: The Herb

Lobelia has a lengthy history of use as an herbal remedy for respiratory conditions such as asthma, bronchitis, pneumonia, and cough. Traditionally, Native Americans smoked lobelia as a treatment for asthma.

Today, some herbalists use lobelia to help clear mucus from the respiratory tract, including the throat, lungs, and bronchial tubes. Additionally, Lobelia is used as part of a comprehensive treatment plan for asthma.

Lobelia is often used to stimulate perspiration to reduce fever; it is also used as an expectorant to expel phlegm in cases of bronchitis and laryngitis. Lobelia also acts to calm the nerves and acts as a mild sedative.

An active alkaloid in Lobelia—lobeline mimics nicotine in the body and is therefore useful as a nicotine substitute for anyone trying to stop smoking. Lobeline does not contain the harmful substances that nicotine does.

Lobelia contains vitamin A, C, and minerals cobalt, copper, iron, lead, manganese, selenium, sodium and sulfur.

Historical Uses:	
Asthma	Bronchitis
Bronchitis	Catarrh
Congestion	Cough
Expectorant	Laryngitis
Nicotine Substitute	Pneumonia

Maca

Plant Parts Used: Root

Maca, also known as Peruvian Ginseng—although it does not belong to the ginseng family—it is used to increase stamina, energy and sexual function in both men and women. In one study, researchers found that Maca may help alleviate sexual dysfunction caused by the use of selective-serotonin re-uptake inhibitors (SSRIs) which are used in the treatment of depression.

In Peru Maca is also sold as a mild laxative due to the fiber content in the herb. It is said to also support the immune system, as well as being used in cases of anemia, menstrual and menopausal disorders. It is also used for memory function and to give clarity to the mind.

Historical Uses:	
Anemia	Erectile Dysfunction
Immune System Support	Impotence
Laxative	Memory

Marjoram

Plant Parts Used: Leaves and Flower Tops

Marjoram is often taken for motion sickness as well as to soothe the digestive tract where it acts as an antispasmodic. For women it is often used in cases of menstrual cramps.

Marjoram can inhibit the growth of the herpes simplex virus which is responsible for cold sores and genital herpes. Due to its calmative and stimulant properties, it is often used in cases of asthma, coughs.

Marjoram contains vitamin A, B1 (Thiamine), B2 (Riboflavin), B12 (Cyanocobalamin), and minerals calcium, iron, magnesium, phosphorus, potassium, silicon, sodium and zinc.

Historical Uses:	
Asthma	Cough
Digestive System Disorders	Herpes Simplex Virus
Menstrual Cramps	

Marshmallow

Plant Parts Used: Root

Marshmallow is a great healing herb. This mucilant herb soothes the kidneys when they are irritated or inflamed. Marshmallow contains volatile oils and tannins that are responsible for its diuretic actions. It is especially helpful in passing kidney stones.

It is also an expectorant which helps remove mucus from the lungs; in addition to difficult to remove phlegm and for helping to relax bronchial tubes where it has a soothing and healing action.

For cases of diarrhea and dysentery it helps reduce inflammation and has a soothing and healing action.

When used externally as a gel it may help the healing process for burns, cuts and wounds. It can be used internally for bronchitis, colds, coughs flu and sore throats.

Marshmallow contains vitamin A, B Complex and minerals iodine, iron and sodium.

Historical Uses:	
Bronchitis	Colds
Cough	Diarrhea
Dysentery	Flu
Helps Expel Kidney Stones	Kidney Support
Lung Infections	

Milk Thistle

Plant Parts Used: Seeds

This natural support to the liver contains a mixture of bioflavo-noids, including silymarin. Milk Thistle strengthens the liver against auto-intoxication and stimulates protein synthesis in liver cells, which generates DNA and RNA.

Milk Thistle has antioxidant properties which help to scavenge free radicals which destroy the body's cells.

Anyone who consumes any amount of alcohol should consider using Milk Thistle, as alcohol residue winds-up in the liver where it forms toxins. Silymarin assists in expelling these toxins and as a result, enhances liver function.

Historical Uses:	
Free Radical Scavenger	Immune System Support
Liver Problems	

Mullein

Plant Parts Used: Leaves, Flowers and Roots

Mullein has both mucilant and astringent properties. Its powerful healing abilities make it useful for healing weak lung tissue and chronic respiratory congestion. It is recommended internally for colds, coughs and sore throat and externally in a warm vinegar compress for hemorrhoids. Because it contains astringent tannins, it is often used to treat cases of diarrhea. It has proven expectorant action that likely arises from saponin compounds in the plant. Scientific studies suggest that the mucilage in mullein protects mucous membranes, preventing cell invasion by viral allergens.

Historical Uses:	
Asthma	Bronchitis
Colds	Congestion
Cough	Diarrhea
Hemorrhoids	Lung Problems
Respiratory System Support	Sore Throat

Myrrh

Plant Parts Used: The Oleo-Gum-Resin from the stem of the tree.

Myrrh originates in the Middle East where it has been used for thousands of years. It is mentioned several times in the Bible. Probably the best known reference concerns the birth of Jesus in Bethlehem *"And when they were come into the house, they saw the young child with Mary his mother, and fell down, and worshipped him: and when they had opened their treasures, they presented unto him gifts; gold, and frankincense and myrrh" (Matthew 2:11)*. You can read the rest of the story in the Bible!

Today Myrrh is used for oral hygiene. As a mouthwash, it contains tannins which have an astringent action on tissue. It also has an anti-inflammatory action in addition to fighting bacteria.

It is also used to treat mouth ulcers and bleeding gums. In addition, herbalists recommend adding powered Myrrh to wounds that have been well cleansed to act as an antiseptic. It can also be mixed with water to use as a gargle to treat a sore throat. It can also be used to treat colds, coughs asthma and congestion of the chest.

Myrrh provides support and strength to the digestive system as well as assisting with waste elimination.

Myrrh is often added to "natural" toothpaste—the best place to look for it is in health food stores—where it is used to help fight the bacteria which cause tooth decay.

Historical Uses:	
Antiseptic	Asthma
Bad Breath	Bleeding Gums
Bronchitis	Colds
Cough	Gum Disease
Mouth Ulcers	Oral Hygiene
Sore Throat	Tooth Decay
Waste Elimination	Wound Healing

Nettle

Plant Parts Used: Leaves, Stem and Root.

We often think of nettle as a nuisance weed that stings—and therefore has to be destroyed at all cost! However it has many uses in herbal medicine. In Germany it is prescribed for circulatory system support and to reduce high blood pressure. Because of its high vitamin C content it is traditionally used to prevent scurvy.

As the plant contains alkaloids which neutralize uric acid, it is used to treat cases of rheumatism. American Indian women drank nettle tea during pregnancy to strengthen the fetus and ease delivery. It was also used by them to stop cases of uterine bleeding after childbirth.

The root of the plant contains tannins which have been used as an enema to shrink hemorrhoids. Nettle can also be used as a tonic to strengthen the whole body.

Nettle is highly nutritious. You can boil or stem the young leaves and eat them as a vegetable. When the stems are boiled, they lose their sting. They can therefore be used in salads.

Nettle contains vitamin A, C, D, E, F, P, and minerals calcium, chromium, copper, iron, manganese, silicon, sodium, sulfur and zinc.

Historical Uses:	
Circulatory System Support	Hemorrhoids
High Blood Pressure	Pregnancy
Purifies the Blood	Rheumatism
Scurvy	Uterine Bleeding

Nopal

Plant Parts Used: Stems, Flowers, Leaf Pads

Nopal or Prickly Peak as it is sometimes called is a cactus which is traditionally used by the Mexicans as a food especially in salads. The nutritional factors in Nopal act in the bowel to prevent fat and excessive sugars from entering the bloodstream. By helping the body maintain balanced blood sugar levels, Nopal aids the body in its battle against obesity. Additionally, it is used as an anti-inflammatory, as a laxative and as a hypoglycemic support for diabetes and gastritis.

In studies, it has also been shown to reduce Low Density Lipoprotein (LDL) cholesterol—the "bad" cholesterol.

Nopal's primary role is focused on supporting the digestive system through the colon, liver and pancreas.

Nopal is a rich source of various nutrients including: all the 9 essential amino acids as well as 8 non-essential amino acids, which makes it an easily digestible form of protein. It also contains vitamin B1 (Thiamine), B2 (Riboflavin), B3 (Niacin), Beta Carotene (which the body converts to vitamin A as it is needed) and C; also the minerals calcium, iron, magnesium, potassium and sodium. In addition, it is also a rich source of mucilage and pectin as well as insoluble plant fiber which is helpful in a weight-loss program, as it gives a feeling of fullness and restricts the urge to food binge.

Historical Uses:	
Anti-Inflammatory	Blood Sugar Imbalance
Cholesterol Reduction	Colon Health
Diabetes	Digestive System Support
Food Cravings	Gastritis
Laxative	Liver Health
Obesity	Pancreas
Weight Loss	

Oatstraw

Plant Parts Used: Stems

Oatstraw is a good source of minerals for nourishing bones, hair, skin and nails. It helps calm the nervous system and can assist in depressive and conditions of exhaustion. When eaten as a food, it can help prevent contagious diseases.

Oatstraw contains vitamin A, B1 (Thiamine), B2 (Riboflavin), E, and minerals calcium, phosphorus and silicon.

Historical Uses:	
Arthritis	Bone Health
Depression	Nails
Nervous Exhaustion	Nervous System Support
Skin Health	

Olive Leaf

Plant Parts Used: Leaves

Olive leaves have been used for centuries to treat cases of fever and malaria. In more recent times researchers have discovered that Olive Leaf contains phytochemicals which strengthen the immune system and are effective against many types of viral pathogens which can cause colds, flu, fungal and yeast infections, as well as bacterial infections and parasitic invasions.

Olive Leaf is also used to support normal blood pressure and cholesterol levels by reducing the effect of Low Density Lipoprotein (LDL) cholesterol that can cause the formation of plaque in the arteries which can result in a heart attack.

Olive Leave is a very effective natural treatment for the Herpes Simplex virus type 1 which causes cold sores, type 2 which is associated with genital herpes and herpes keratitis which is quite serious as it causes inflammation of the cornea in the eye.

Studies suggest that Olive Leaf may have anti-inflammatory properties which would make it useful as a treatment for inflammation of the lungs and respiratory tract as well as osteoarthritis and rheumatoid arthritis.

Historical Uses:	
Anti-Inflammatory	Candida Yeast Infections
Cholesterol Reduction	Colds
Fever	Flu
Herpes Simplex Virus	High Blood Pressure
Lung Support	Malaria
Osteoarthritis	Parasites
Respiratory System Support	Rheumatoid Arthritis
Urinary System Support	

Oregon Grape

Plant Parts Used: Root

Oregon Grape is mainly used as a blood cleanser where there are toxins in the blood which cause skin diseases such as eczema, psoriasis, herpes and acne. It also supports thyroid function, and is in fact a tonic for all the glandular system.

It supports a healthy liver and gall bladder by increasing bile flow, and as it has antibacterial properties it is often used to treat a candida yeast overgrowth, diarrhea, parasites and urinary tract infections.

Historical Uses:	
Acne	Blood Cleanser
Candida Yeast Infections	Constipation
Diarrhea	Eczema
Gall Bladder Support	Herpes Simplex Virus
Liver Health	Parasites
Psoriasis	Urinary Tract Infections

Oregano

Plant Parts Used: Leaves and Stems

Oregano is often thought of as seasoning on pizza—but it is used for far more than that.

Available in either enteric coated (meaning it will burst in the body where it is supposed to), or in liquid form, oregano possesses anti-inflammatory antiviral and anti-fungal properties which makes it especially useful for eradicating candida yeast.

It also supports the digestive system by soothing the smooth muscle lining of the digestive tract. Oregano also has uses for expelling worms.

Oils in Oregano act to expel phlegm—by loosening it so that it can be expectorated more easily. It is also used for colds, flu and congestion of the chest.

Historical Uses:	
Candida Yeast Infections	Colds
Congestion	Digestive System Support
Flu	Inflammatory Conditions
Worms	

Papaya

Plant Parts Used: Fruit

Although not an herb, Papaya contains papain—a proteolytic enzyme that aids in the digestion of proteins.

We grow Papaya trees in our garden in Florida, and it is nice to go and pick the fruit for breakfast.

Papaya has a soothing effect in the stomach where it has been used to help prevent ulcers from forming. When the seeds are mixed with honey, they help to expel intestinal worms. It is also an excellent blood clotting agent

Papaya contains vitamin A, B, C, D, E, G, K, and minerals calcium, iron, magnesium phosphorus, potassium and sodium.

Historical Uses:	
Digestive System Support	For Blood Clotting
Intestinal Worms	Protein Digestion

Parsley

Plant Parts Used: Leaves, Seeds

Parsley is probably one of the best known herbs as it is used in culinary dishes as well as for medicinal uses. It comes in a variety of different "leaf types", from feather like to curled to flat. The flat leafed variety is most often used for medicinal purposes.

It is used to treat urinary tract infections, indigestion, to relieve the effects of gas and as a digestive aid. Additionally, as it has a high chlorophyll content, it is a natural body deodorizer and eradicates bad breath.

In Germany, a tea made from Parsley Seeds is prescribed to treat high blood pressure due to its diuretic action.

A recent study determined that Parsley limits the secretion of histamine—a chemical produced by the body that causes allergy symptoms, especially hay fever.

Parsley contains vitamin A, B1 (Thiamine), B2 (Riboflavin), C and minerals calcium, cobalt, copper, potassium, silicon, sodium and sulfur.

Historical Uses:	
Bad Breath	Bloating
Body Deodorizer	Digestive System Support
Gas	Hay Fever
High Blood Pressure	Indigestion
Urinary Tract Infections	

Passion Flower

Plant Parts Used: Leaves

A natural sedative, passionflower will help you sleep without leaving a groggy feeling the next morning. It is beneficial for calming the nervous system, and for stress conditions.

Passion Flower slows the breakdown of neurotransmitters which pass chemical messages between the body's cells, as well as working with certain enzymes. It also assists in calming an irritable bowel, as well as killing certain bacteria—especially those that cause eye irritation.

Several studies show that it relieves pain as well as having the ability to kill and eradicate disease causing bacteria, fungi and mold.

Historical Uses:	
Eye Bacteria	Eye Irritation
Fever	Insomnia
Irritable Bowel Syndrome (IBS)	Kills Bacteria
Kills Fungi	Kills Mold
Nervous System Support	Relieves Pain
Stress	Vision Problems

Pau D'Arco

Plant Parts Used: Outer and Inner Bark

Pau D'Arco is a tree which is native to Central and South American rain forests. It contains a chemical called lapachol, which may provide nutritional support to the immune system. It is commonly used against many conditions of unwanted growth, including fungi, yeast and tumors as well as fungal infections, arthritis, ulcers and diabetes.

Pau D'Arco is also used to reduce inflammation, treat infections and support the digestive system. Other uses include: flushing toxins from the body and for circulatory system support to reduce high blood pressure and as a protector against heart disease.

It is also used to treat lupus, osteomyelitis, Parkinson's disease, psoriasis and as a pain reliever. The bark can be used externally when boiled as a poultice or when the liquid is strained it can be used to treat skin inflammation as well as hemorrhoids, eczema, and wounds.

Historically, it has also been used to remedy the side effects of some antibiotics.

It is available as a capsule, tablet or as a lotion. It can also be made into a tea.

Historical Uses:	
Antibiotic Side Effects	Arthritis
Auto Immune Conditions	Body Cleanse
Candida Yeast Infections	Circulatory System Support
Colds	Diabetes
Eczema	Flu
Immune System Support	Lupus
Pain Relief	Parkinson's Disease
Psoriasis	Skin Inflammation
Tumors	Ulcers

Pennyroyal

Plant Parts Used: Leaves and Flower Tops

A member of the mint family, Pennyroyal contains a chemical (pulegone) within its oil that is often used as an insect repellent—especially against mosquitoes, fleas, gnats, flies and ticks. In fact several natural insect killers contain the oil from Pennyroyal.

Pennyroyal is also used as a decongestant and cough remedy due to its strong aromatic smell, which acts as a decongestant. It also supports the digestive system in cases of stomach discomfort and bloating where it will expel gas.

Historical Uses:	
Cough	Decongestant
Digestive System Support	Expels Gas
Insect repellent	

Peppermint

Plant Parts Used: Leaves, Oil

Peppermint—a member of the mint family is closely related to spearmint and water mint. Peppermint Oil stimulates the production of digestive fluids. It also eradicates bad breath and helps settle an upset stomach.

Peppermint oil has been used to support the digestive system and to treat irritable bowel syndrome, and for indigestion. It is often used for motion sickness.

If purchased in liquid form as an oil, then only tiny drops should be applied to water, otherwise it will be too strong.

Peppermint contains vitamin A, B6 (Pyridoxine), B12 (Cyanocobalamin), C, D, and minerals calcium, iron, magnesium, potassium and sodium.

Historical Uses	
Bad Breath	Colds
Cough	Digestive System Support
Gas	Indigestion
Motion Sickness	Nausea
Respiratory Infections	Sinus Infections
Sore Throat (Gargle)	Stomach Upset

Psyllium

Plant Parts Used: Seeds

Psyllium is an excellent source of fiber—and is especially useful for those individuals who suffer from celiac disease as it contains no gluten. It is important to drink plenty of water with Psyllium as this helps it work better.

Psyllium acts as a sponge in the colon, soaking up toxins which can then be eliminated. It is non-irritating to the mucus membranes in the intestinal tract, but instead, strengthens and tones them.

Historical Uses:	
Colitis	Colon Cleansing
Constipation	Diverticulitis
Reduces Inflammation	Toxic Waste Removal

Pumpkin

Plant Parts Used: Seeds

Pumpkin Seeds have powerful antioxidant properties due to its vitamin E content. However, it does not contain just one form of vitamin E, but several. This is what makes it so powerful. In addition, it contains the antioxidant mineral zine, which adds to its potency.

One of the best tasting of all the anti-parasite herbal products. The seeds can be eaten as a snack. In fact they taste so good that you cannot eat enough of them. Pumpkin Seeds are very effective against tapeworms as well as other types of parasites.

Recent studies also suggest that Pumpkin Seeds can also be of benefit in regulating insulin, and in the prevention of some of the unwanted side effects of diabetes that affect kidney function. In addition, a decrease in oxidative stress has played a significant role in health improvement for those who have diabetes.

Men can benefit from Pumpkin Seeds due to the high concentration of zinc which is important for prostate health as a man ages. The biggest concentration of zinc is found in the prostate gland. In addition to zinc, Pumpkin Seeds contain various oils which are helpful in treating benign prostatic hyperplasia (BPH), or to give it its more common name—enlarged prostate.

Pumpkin Seeds contain vitamin E and minerals copper, iron, magnesium, manganese, phosphorus and zinc. They are also a good source of protein.

Pumpkin Seeds are a good source of alpha linolenic acid (ALA)—a plant based omega-3 essential fatty acid—which are essential for good health.

Historical Uses:	
Anti-Parasitic	Diabetes
Heart Health	Liver Health
Oxidative Stress	Parasites
Prostate Health	Restful Sleep
Worms	

Pygeum

Plant Parts Used: Bark

Obtained from the bark of a tree in Africa, Pygeum is used to prevent and relieve benign prostatic hyperplasia (BPH), or to give it its more common name—enlarged prostate. It contains anti-inflammatory phytosterol compounds in addition to triterpenoid compounds which have an anti-swelling effect.

Historical Uses	
Benign Prostatic Hyperplasia (BPH)	Nocturnal Urinary Frequency
Prostate Inflammation	Sexual Dysfunction
Urinary System Disorders (Men)	

Red Clover

Plant Parts Used: Flower Tops

Red Clover has been cultivated as forage since prehistoric times. In more recent times, Red Clover has been used as a cancer treatment for non-estrogen dependent cancers. Researchers from the National Cancer Institute (NCI) have identified four anti tumor compounds in Red Clover. They also discovered that a high concentration of tocopherol—a form of the antioxidant vitamin E was also present in the plant.

In addition, studies show that Red Clover acts like the female sex hormone estrogen, which means it, may alleviate menopausal symptoms. Red Clover also supports the nervous system in cases of nervous exhaustion.

Red Clover contains vitamin A, B Complex, C, F, P, and minerals calcium, cobalt, copper, magnesium, manganese, nickel, selenium, sodium and tin.

Historic Uses:	
Cancer (Non-Estrogen Related)	Menopause
Nervous Exhaustion	Nervous System Support

Red Raspberry

Plant Parts Used: Leaves, Fruit

A common backyard fruit bush, this herb is renowned for its nutritional support of the female reproductive system. Red Raspberry is known to nourish and strengthen the uterus. In addition, Raspberry Leaves contain tannins which make it a useful treatment in cases of diarrhea.

Red Raspberry contains vitamin A, B3 (Niacin), C, D, E, F, G and minerals calcium, iron, manganese, and phosphorus.

Historical Uses:	
Colds	Constipation
Diarrhea	Digestive System Support
Female Reproductive System	Fever
Flu	

Rosemary

Plant Parts Used: Leaves

Rosemary, a member of the mint family is an excellent tonic and improves circulation and supports the nervous system as well as enhancing the memory. It complements other members of the mint family in addition to lavender and other herbs. It can be used in various forms. For example:

Rosemary Leaf Extract

Rosemary Leaf Extract as well as being excellent for the nervous system, it also supports the digestive system where problems arise due to emotional stress. In addition, it is also an excellent antibacterial and has astringent properties.

Rosemary Tea

Rosemary Tea has been drunk for centuries to ease the effects of headaches as well as improving circulation and neutralizing some of the effects of memory loss. It can help when working long hours or studying to help keep the mind focused on the task at hand. Like Rosemary Leaf Extract, it is also beneficial for the digestive system. Cold rosemary tea can be used as an antibacterial mouth wash.

Historical Uses:	
Bad Breath	Circulatory System Support
Digestive System Support	Emotional Stress
Headaches	Memory Loss
Mouthwash	Nervous System Support

Saffron

Plant Parts Used: Stigmas within the flowers

Spain is the world's leading exporter of Saffron which was introduced into the country in the 8th century by the Arabs. It helps protect against heart disease by reducing cholesterol through deactivating uric acid build-up. In parts of Spain where Saffron is grown and eaten on a daily basis, there are very few instances of heart disease.

In Indian Ayurvedic medicine Saffron is used to stimulate the circulatory system, and is used for kidney and liver conditions.

Saffron contains vitamin A, B12 (Cyanocobalamin), and minerals calcium, phosphorus, potassium, and sodium.

Historical Uses:	
Bronchitis	Circulatory System Support
Digestive System Support	Gas
Headaches	Kidney Problems
Liver Problems	Prevents Heart Disease
Reduces Cholesterol	

Sage

Plant Parts Used: Leaves

This aromatic herb is probably best known at Thanksgiving for being used in turkey stuffing. However, culinary uses aside; it is also an important herb in the herbal medicine chest.

It has been used historically as an antiperspirant and to reduce fevers. Scientific studies have determined that Sage will cut perspiration by up to 50 per cent approximately two hours after ingestion. This is why it proved so useful to reduce sweating from fever.

Sage has been used as a treatment for wound healing due to its anti-bacterial activity. It is also a potent antioxidant and as such it has been used to preserve meat. In fact, it is often used to inhibit bacteria growth in hamburger meat prior to the meat being grilled on a barbecue. Food hygiene is an important consideration especially when meat may be left out for extended periods of time in a warm sunny environment. Bacteria in meat can cause stomach upsets as well as food poisoning.

Sage steeped in warm water can be used as a gargle for sore throat and tonsillitis. A study conducted in Germany determined that Sage made into an infusion and consumed on an empty stomach can reduce blood sugar levels in diabetics.

Historical Uses:	
Anti-Perspirant	Bacteria
Bleeding Gums	Diabetes
Diarrhea	Digestive System Support
Intestinal System Support	Reduce Sweating from Fever
Urinary Tract Infections	Wound Healing

Sarsaparilla

Plant Parts Used: Root

Historically Sarsaparilla was used as a blood purifier to treat syphilis—which was quite common in 19th century America. In more recent times it has been used to treat colds, cough, fever and gout.

Sarsaparilla supports the glandular system and contains the male hormone testosterone, as well as progesterone—a female hormone produced in the ovaries.

Sarsaparilla contains vitamin A, B Complex, C, D and minerals copper, iodine, iron, manganese, silicon, sodium, sulfur and zinc.

Historical Uses:	
Blood Purifier	Colds
Cough	Fever
Glandular System Support	Gout
Syphilis	

Saw Palmetto

Plant Parts Used: Fruit

Saw Palmetto has an influence on all glandular tissue therefore it is a useful herb for all wasting diseases, and is used for diseases of the reproductive glands. It is also used to treat benign prostatic hyperplasia (BPH). BPH is a male condition which includes frequent urination, difficulty in fulfilling the urge to urinate, dribbling after urination, a weak urinary stream, and finally, waking up several times at night to urinate.

Historical Uses:	
Benign Prostatic Hyperplasia (BPH)	Glandular System Diseases
Glandular System Support	Male Prostate
Reproductive Glands	Urinary System Disorders (Men)

Skullcap

Plant Parts Used: Leaves

Skullcap is a member of the mint family and is traditionally used as a nerve tonic as well as a tranquilizer and sedative for relieving anxiety and insomnia. In addition it relieves nervous exhaustion and supports the nervous system.

Historical Uses:	
Anxiety	Insomnia
Nervous System Support	Sedative
Stress	Tranquilizer

Shepherds Purse

Plant Parts Used: Leaves and Flower Tops

Shepherds Purse contains compounds that assist in blood clotting—and therefore this herb is useful to stop bleeding in wounds. It is also used to treat hemorrhoids due to its astringent action.

It is also used to constrict blood vessels and is therefore useful to control either high or low blood pressure as well as heart function.

Shepherds Purse contains vitamin C, E, K and minerals calcium, iron, magnesium, potassium, sodium, sulfur, tin and zinc.

Historical Uses:	
Blood Clotting	Heart Action
High Blood Pressure	Low Blood Pressure
Wound Healing	

Slippery Elm

Plant Parts Used: Inner Bark

Slippery Elm is very soothing to inflamed tissue—especially in the gastrointestinal tract—and as a result, is excellent for tissue healing. It is easily digested and has good laxative properties. It helps neutralize acidity in the stomach and soaks-up foul gases.

Slippery Elm provides glandular system support by assisting the adrenal glands in performing their important functions.

Slippery Elm has been used historically for wound healing. The herb bark has a cell-like structure which expands when mixed with liquid. When applied to a cleaned wound, it has the effect of forming an herbal seal, which helps keep bacteria out and encourages healing.

Slippery Elm contains vitamin E, F, K, P and minerals calcium, copper, iodine, iron, phosphorus, potassium, selenium, sodium and zinc.

Historical Uses:	
Adrenal Gland Support	Digestive System Support
Glandular System Support	Inflammation
Intestinal System Support	Laxative
Wound Healing	

St. John's Wort

Plant Parts Used: Leaves and Flowers

St John's Wort has been used as an herbal medicine for over 2,000 years—mainly for healing wounds.

This popular herb has gained national attention for its ability to alleviate mild to moderate depression. It contains an active constituent, hypericin, which appears to prolong the activity of serotonin (a neurotransmitter) in the brain. St. John's Wort may also lengthen the performance of dopamine and norepinephrine, two brain chemicals that are linked to depression. In Europe, many doctors prescribe this herb instead of prescription antidepressant drugs.

Note! You can find further details on Stress and Depression by reading my book "An Easy Way to Understand Stress and Depression", which is available from the Kindle Store, or there is a download printable version available at www.wisdomforlifemedia.com.

Recent studies have determined that St John's Wort has a positive effect against several virus strains including HIV which causes AIDS. Since the study, various AIDS patients have reported encouraging outcomes by taking the herb. More studies are underway to further understand the anti-viral mechanism in this herb.

Historical Uses:	
AIDS	Anti-Viral
Anxiety	Bed Wetting
Depression	HIV
Nervous System Support	Wound Healing

Thyme

Plant Parts Used: Leaves and Flower Tops

Thyme is often thought of as an herb that is used in the kitchen along with sage, parsley and rosemary. However, it has important medicinal uses, and is often included in over-the-counter mouthwashes and decongestants.

Thyme contains aromatic oil which is an antispasmodic, and is used for digestive problems—by relaxing the smooth muscle tissue of the gastrointestinal tract, as well as being useful for treating bacterial and viral infections. As an expectorant, it is also used for cough—to loosen and expel phlegm, as well as for laryngitis, sore throat, whooping cough and nervous system disorders.

Additionally, it is used externally as an antiseptic for treating wounds which aids healing.

Thyme contains vitamin B Complex, C, E and minerals iodine, silicone, sodium and sulfur.

Historical Uses:	
Antiseptic	Bacteria Infections
Colds	Cough
Digestive System Disorders	Intestinal System Disorders
Laryngitis	Phlegm
Sore Throat	Virus
Whooping Cough	Wound Healing

Una de Gato (Cats Claw)

Plant Parts Used: Bark

The bark of a vine from the Peruvian rainforests in South America, where it has been used for centuries, by local natives, to treat a variety of medical conditions. Una de Gato provides beneficial alkaloids to stimulate the immune system. It is used as a cancer therapy to reduce the side effects of chemotherapy. It is also used as an anti-inflammatory for all types of arthritis.

Una de Gato is also used as a bowel and stomach protector and cleanser, and to treat ulcerative colitis, Crohn's disease, diverticulitis and irritable bowel syndrome (IBS) as well as stomach ulcers.

Una de Gato is rich in proanthocyanidins—antioxidants which fight free radical damage, and help strengthen the circulatory system, as well as decrease inflammation and the production of histamine and offers protection to collagen—the main component of connective tissues.

One controlled study confirmed the existence of various alkaloids in Una de Gato which fight against the HIV virus. Participants in the study with HIV achieved a reduction in the symptoms of HIV during their first year of treatment.

Una de Gato is an excellent general body tonic to tone and protect all body systems. It is often taken in capsule form.

Historical Uses:	
Anti-Inflammatory	Antioxidant
Chemotherapy Effects	Circulatory System Support
Collagen Protection	Crohn's Disease
Diverticulitis	HIV
Immune System Support	Irritable Bowel Syndrome (IBS)
Reduces Histamine	Stomach Ulcers
Ulcerative Colitis	

Uva Ursi

Plant Parts Used: Leaves

Uva Ursi is used to treat cystitis – inflammation of the urinary tract. The main component of Uva Ursi is arbutin. Arbutin is absorbed in the stomach where it is converted into a substance with antimicrobial, astringent and antimicrobial properties.

Arbutin's main purpose is to soothe irritation and reduce inflammation during urination, as well as to fight infections in the urinary tract.

It is important for the urine to be alkaline for Uva Ursi to work properly. The acid / alkaline balance (pH) can be determined by using a litmus paper test strip. If the urine is too acidic then it can be brought to an alkaline state by the use of alkalizing agents such as calcium, magnesium supplements, chlorophyll in liquid form (chlorophyll is derived from alfalfa), and by eating alkalizing foods such as tomatoes, and the majority of fruits and vegetables. This is by no means a complete list. Note. While most citrus fruits are acidic, when they have been digested they are alkaline forming.

Acidic foods to avoid would be mainly beef, pork, lamb, butter, peanut butter, and many more. There are some excellent acid / alkaline food lists available on the Internet. Just type "acid alkaline food lists" into your search engine.

Uva Ursi also contains Allantoin which may help speed-up the healing of wounds. Several over the counter skin creams designed for skin infections also contain Allantoin as the active ingredient. Uva Ursi also contains tannins which have an astringent effect which help treat diarrhea.

Historical Uses:	
Bed Wetting	Cystitis
Diarrhea	Kidney Infections
Urinary System Support	Urinary Tract Inflammation
Wound Healing	

Valerian

Plant Parts Used: Root

Valerian Root—a natural plant calcium – is often used as a pain killer. It has been used for centuries to treat anxiety and insomnia, and is best taken before bedtime. It provides excellent support for the nervous system, and in addition, provides support for the structural system in cases of muscle spasms.

Valerian contains minerals copper, magnesium, potassium and zinc.

Historical Uses:	
Anxiety	Insomnia
Muscle Spasms	Pain Relief

Violet

Plant Parts Used: Leaves and Flowers

Violet Leaf and flowers has antifungal properties in addition to being a diuretic and laxative. It can be used externally as well as internally for a variety of conditions including: abscesses, boils, sore Throat and tumors. It is also used to treat internal ulcers.

Violet is a good source of vitamin C and beta carotene (which the body converts to vitamin A as needed).

Historical Uses:	
Abscesses	Boils
Sore Throat	Tumors
Ulcers	

White Willow

Plant Parts Used: Bark

The use of White Willow Bark goes back to the time of Hippocrates. This Greek physician wrote about the medicinal benefits of White Willow Bark in the 5th century B.C.

However, it was in 1829 that scientists in Europe identified salicin as being the active ingredient in the bark, which is converted in the body to salicylic acid.

It was used as a popular remedy for the relief of pain in such conditions as inflammation, fever, joint pain and osteoarthritis.

Extracting salicin from herbs was a time consuming process, so in 1852, German scientists developed a synthetic form of salicylic acid. Unfortunately this had a tendency to cause stomach ulcers and bleeding.

Eventually the German company Bayer developed a synthetic version being less harsh which they called acetylsalicylic acid (ASA). This was then manufactured under the trade name aspirin. Today, low dose soluble aspirin is recommended by doctors to reduce a person's risk of a heart attack or stroke by 50 percent. However, aspirin still has the stigma of being associated with causing stomach bleeding and irritating the stomach lining.

Many people prefer White Willow Bark to aspirin because it does not irritate the stomach lining. Researchers have identified a possible reason for this in that salicin found naturally in white willow bark is only converted to the acid form after it is absorbed by the stomach.

Any health condition such as fever, inflammation, pain you would use aspirin for, you could try White Willow instead. In cases of women's health, salicin suppresses the actions of prostaglandins which are associated with menstrual cramps

Historical Uses:	
Fever	Headaches
Inflammation	Menstrual Cramps
Pain	

Wild Cherry

Plant Parts Used: Inner Bark

Wild Cherry contains a volatile oil which makes it a useful expectorant in cases of excess catarrh, phlegm and bronchitis, colds, cough and asthma. It also has a mild sedative action.

Wild Cherry Supports the digestive system, and is often used as a tonic after an illness to benefit all the body systems.

Historical Uses:	
Asthma	Bronchitis
Colds	Cough
Digestive System Support	Sedative
Tranquilizer	

Wild Yam

Plant Parts Used: Root

Wild Yam supports the glandular system, and is used by pregnant women as a treatment for nausea, to help reduce cramps in later stages of pregnancy, and to help prevent a miscarriage.

It helps support the nervous system and helps reduce the pain associated with gallstones.

Historical Uses:	
Gallstones	Glandular System Support
Miscarriages	Nervous System Support

Witch Hazel

Plant Parts Used: Leaves and Bark

Witch Hazel has excellent anti-inflammatory and antiseptic properties. As it has a high flavonoid content, this helps to heal damaged blood vessels. It is also an astringent herb and is widely used to treat bruises, burns, cuts, hemorrhoids, inflammation, scalds and sore muscles.

It is recommended as a gargle for a sore throat and for mouth sores. It can be used internally to relieve symptoms of diarrhea.

Witch Hazel contains vitamin C, E, K, P and minerals copper, iodine, manganese, selenium and zinc.

Historical Uses:	
Bruises	Burns
Cuts	Diarrhea
Gargle	Hemorrhoids
Inflammation	Mouth Sores
Scalds	Sore Muscles
Sore Throat	

Yarrow

Plant Parts Used: Leaves, Stem, Flower

Yarrow has many uses in Herbal Medicine. It is often used for wound healing due to the various chemicals contained within the plant. It is used as an antiseptic to kill bacteria, for blood clotting, and as an anti-inflammatory and pain reliever.

Yarrow also supports the digestive system as it contains a chemical similar to chamomile which helps relax the smooth muscle tissue of the digestive tract.

It helps support the glandular system, and has a useful role to play as a sedative.

Yarrow contains vitamin A, C, E, F, K and minerals copper, iodine, iron, manganese, and potassium.

Historical Uses:	
Anti-Inflammatory	Antiseptic
Bacteria Infections	Blood Clotting
Digestive System Support	Glandular System Support
Sedative	Wound Healing

Yellow Dock

Plant Parts Used: Root

Yellow Dock assists with elimination and is one of the best blood builders available in the herbal medicine chest. It has astringent properties and as such, is used to treat skin conditions.

Due to its high iron content, it is used to treat cases of anemia. It nurtures the liver and spleen, and as a result, is used to treat conditions associated with the lymphatic system as well as jaundice.

Yellow Dock contains vitamin A, C and minerals iron, manganese and nickel.

Historical Uses:	
Anemia	Blood Building
Blood Purifier	Elimination
Jaundice	Liver
Lymphatic System	Skin Conditions
Spleen	

Yerba Mate

Plant Parts Used: Leaves and Stems

Yerba Mate is a tree—a member of the holly family—that grows in the rainforests of Argentina, Brazil and Paraguay.

The leaves naturally contain 24 vitamins and minerals, 15 amino acids, as well as antioxidant activity. Yerba mate contains caffeine (but unlike caffeine containing plants, Yerba Mate does not cause the jitters or shakes,) theophylline, and theobromine, which are stimulants that are also found in tea, coffee and chocolate.

Yerba Mate is used to boost energy and stamina, as an aid to elimination and stimulates clarity and focus. It is also used in weight loss programs that incorporate a balanced diet and exercise. It is also used to treat asthma and various allergies.

Yerba Mate is usually made into a tea by pouring hot water on to the leaves, and then it is left for 10 minutes before straining.

Yerba Mate contains vitamin A, B1 (Thiamine), B2 (Riboflavin), B3 (Niacin) B5 (Pantothenic Acid), B Complex, C, E, and minerals calcium, iron, magnesium, manganese, phosphorus, potassium, selenium and zinc. Additions compounds include: chlorophyll, fatty acids, flavonoids, inositol, polyphenols, tannins and 15 amino acids.

Historical Uses:	
Allergies	Asthma
Clarity	Constipation
Elimination	Energy
Focus	Stamina
Weight Loss	

Yerba Santa

Plant Parts Used: Leaves

Yerba Santa is best known as a treatment for bronchial congestion in the chest area, due to its decongestant action. It also supports the digestive system by promoting digestive secretions.

Historical Uses:	
Bronchial Congestion	Bronchitis
Catarrh	Colds
Cough	Digestive System Support
Fever	

Yohimbe

Plant Parts Used: Bark

A native to the Congo, Cameroon, Nigeria, and Gabon, Yohimbe is used to prevent depression as it inhibits mono-amine oxidase (MAO). Additionally it is used to treat erectile dysfunction either as a single herb, or in combination with other herbs. It also helps offset sexual side effects of medications that are being taken for depression.

Yohimbe contains a chemical yohimbine which has the ability to increase blood flow and increase nerve transmissions to the penis or vagina.

Yohimbe is also used to control high or low blood pressure, as part of a weight loss program, diabetes, chest pains and nervous system problems. Body builders and athletes also use Yohimbe to help enhance performance in their chosen sport.

Historical Uses:	
Athletic Uses	Body Building
Chest Pains	Depression
Diabetes	Erectile Dysfunction
High Blood Pressure	Impotence
Low Blood Pressure	Nervous System Disorders
Weight Loss Programs	

Yucca

Plant Parts Used: Root

Yucca Root is high in fiber content and as such, is an excellent herb for digestive and intestinal problems. It can rid the body of undigested waste toxins which reside in the colon and cause foul smelling gas.

Historically, Yucca Root has been used as an anti-inflammatory and laxative agent that purges toxins from joints which if left untreated, can cause inflammation that then leads to joint problems such as arthritis. Yucca is also effective at eliminating toxins from the blood, kidneys, liver and lymph.

Yucca contains vitamin A, B Complex, C and minerals calcium, copper, iron, manganese, phosphorus and potassium.

Historical Uses:	
Arthritis	Blood Purifier
Digestive System Disorders	Inflammation
Intestinal System Disorders	Laxative
Toxic Waste Removal	

Consult Your Doctor or a Naturopathic Doctor

In the A-Z of Herbs section I have given a short description of various herbal products that have been used historically by herbalists and naturopaths for many years, but no suggested dosage requirements, or contra-indications.

The reason for this is that everyone is different. One person may need more of a particular product than the next person. Also, a particular product may suit one person, but not another.

Therefore I feel it is extremely important that you consult your doctor or a naturopathic doctor before commencing any supplement or herbal program, or changing your diet.

Additionally, you may be taking prescription medications for various health conditions which will, or could, have a negative impact on your health if you introduce vitamin or mineral supplements or a herbal program. Never take chances with your health.

I know that many doctors are not supportive of using a natural traditional route for health care. If your doctor feels this way and you would like to consider a more natural approach, then change your doctor and find one who is more supportive to your requirements.

About The Author

Brian B Jacques started in business at a young age, and over the ensuing years, he has developed several very successful businesses. But his main interest for the past 35 years has been in natural health research and publishing.

Brian has presented seminars worldwide on such diverse subjects as Health Related issues, Motivation and Personal Development. In addition he has written numerous books, newsletters and articles on these subjects.

His very popular series of Mini Health Books has circulated widely around the world, and many more titles are in preparation.

Brian is a highly motivated individual, so much so that in 1985 he received a UK Industrial Society award for his work in the Motivation and Personal Development fields.

Brian has the following mottos:

- If something does not work out for you, then don't give up, but keep trying, trying, trying until finally you succeed.
- Success or failure in any endeavor is in your own hands.

Brian was born in the UK and lives with his wife in Florida, USA.

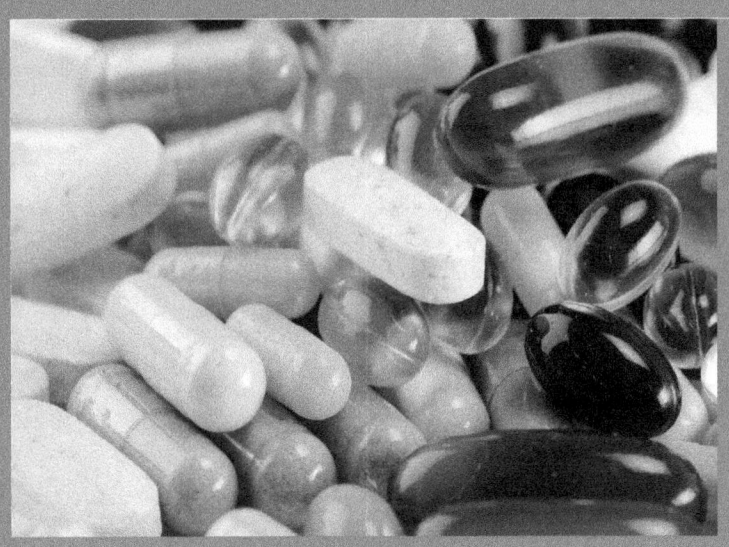

Index of Health Conditions

A

Abdominal Aches 47
Abscesses 24, 114
Aches 39
Acne 19, 31, 60, 88
Adrenal Gland Support 20, 76, 108
AIDS 109
Alcohol Withdrawal 73
Allergies 17, 31, 62, 73, 121
Anemia 17, 36, 62, 72, 78, 120
Angina 63
Anti-bacterial 55
Anti-biotic - natural penicillin 55
Antibiotic Side Effects 93
Anti-Cancer Properties 40
Anti-Inflammatory 85, 87, 111, 119
Antioxidant 111
Anti-Parasitic 97
Anti-Perspirant 103
Antiseptic 51, 83, 110, 119
Anti-Viral 55, 109
Anxiety 37, 38, 65, 71, 74, 75, 106, 109, 113
Aphrodisiac 59
Appetite Stimulant 17, 28, 57, 59, 64
Appetite Suppressant 54, 62
Arteriosclerosis 40, 55, 63
Arthritis 17, 26, 28, 29, 30, 31, 33, 38, 39, 48, 53, 55, 56, 57, 70, 72, 86, 93, 124
Asthma 27, 31, 49, 50, 55, 57, 72, 77, 79, 82, 83, 116, 121
Atherosclerosis 32
Athletes Foot 55
Athletic Uses 123
Auto Immune Conditions 93
Ayurvedic Medicine 61, 62

B

Bacteria 103
Bacterial Infections 18, 28, 55, 57, 64, 70, 110, 119
Bad Breath 17, 39, 41, 83, 91, 95, 101

Balances Blood Sugar Levels 24
Balances Female Hormones 45
Balances Hormones 23, 25
Bed wetting 29
Bed Wetting 29, 67, 109, 112
Benign Prostatic Hyperplasia (BPH) 68, 98, 105
Bites 48
Bladder Control 27
Bladder infection 26
Bleeding 30, 33, 43
Bleeding Gums 22, 83, 103
Bloating 75, 91
Blood Building 120
Blood Circulation 25, 61
Blood Cleanser 20, 33, 39, 40, 72, 88
Blood Clots 47
Blood Clotting 90, 107, 119
Blood poisoning 55
Blood Pressure (Equalizers) 33
Blood Pressure (Low) 107, 123
Blood Purifier 17, 18, 31, 104, 120, 124
Blood Strengthener 56
Blood Sugar Imbalance 70, 85
Blood Sugar Levels 62
Blood Thinner 21
Blood Vessels 21
Body Building 123
Body Cleanse 93
Body Deodorizer 91
Boils 31, 40, 114
Bone Health 86
Bowel Function 30
Bowel Problems 17
Brain 61
Brain (Blood Circulation) 32
Breast Problems 69
Brittle Nails 67
Broken Bones 43
Bronchial Congestion 122
Bronchitis 27, 28, 31, 33, 42, 49, 50, 52, 57, 66, 77, 80, 82, 83, 102, 116, 122

Bruises 61, 118
Burns 33, 40, 43, 51, 118
Bursitis 17

C

Cancer 48, 59
Cancer Fighter 39
Cancer (Non-Estrogen Related) 99
Candida Yeast Infections 38, 46, 48, 72, 87, 88, 89, 93
Carbohydrate Reduction 54
Catarrh 20, 27, 28, 35, 42, 50, 51, 53, 77, 122
Chemical Toxins 59
Chemotherapy Effects 111
Chest Conditions 42
Chest Pains 123
Chest & Throat Congestion 27
Childbirth 31
Chills 28
Cholesterol Reduction 32, 53, 59, 62, 63, 85, 87, 102
Chronic Bronchitis 36
Circulatory System 61
Circulatory System Disorders 64, 67
Circulatory System Support 21, 31, 32, 33, 36, 46, 47, 56, 58, 84, 93, 101, 102, 111
Clarity 121
Cleanses the Kidneys 17
Cold 66
Cold Hands and Feet 21
Colds 19, 20, 27, 28, 33, 34, 36, 38, 42, 48, 49, 51, 53, 57, 64, 69, 73, 80, 82, 83, 87, 89, 93, 95, 100, 104, 110, 116, 122
Cold Sores 69, 75, 76
Colic 26, 34, 36, 52, 75
Colitis 24, 38, 96
Collagen Protection 111
Colon Cleansing 35, 96
Colon Health 27, 85
Congested Sinuses 49
Congestion 33, 52, 77, 82, 89
Congestive Heart Failure 63
Constipation 24, 25, 28, 30, 35, 40, 62, 88, 96, 100, 121
Consumption 27

Convulsions 26, 27, 36
Cough 27, 35, 36, 42, 52, 53, 57, 62, 66, 69, 72, 77, 79, 80, 82, 83, 94, 95,
      104, 110, 116, 122
Cramps 23, 25, 26, 46, 47
Crohn's Disease 111
Croup 35
Cuts 118
Cystitis 29, 112

D

Dandruff 31
Decongestant 55, 94
Depression 86, 109, 123
Detoxify Poisons 46
Diabetes 26, 33, 37, 59, 62, 72, 85, 93, 97, 103, 123
Diarrhea 20, 21, 22, 36, 57, 80, 82, 88, 100, 103, 112, 118
Digestion 17, 34, 35, 36
Digestive System 72
Digestive System Disorders 17, 43, 49, 69, 75, 79, 110, 124
Digestive System Support 25, 38, 41, 50, 52, 56, 57, 60, 65, 85, 89, 90, 91,
      94, 95, 100, 101, 102, 103, 108, 116, 119, 122
Diuretic 64
Diverticulitis 96, 111
Dizziness 58
Dropsy 37
Dysentery 20, 22, 80
Dyspepsia 35

E

Earache 27
Ear Problems 60
Eczema 31, 38, 48, 60, 66, 72, 88, 93
Edema 68
Effects of Radiation 59
Elephantitis 61
Elimination 120, 121
Emotional Stress 101
Energy 59, 72, 76, 121
Enhances Memory Function 25
Enlarged Heart 63
Epilepsy 26, 61

Equalizers Blood Pressure 33
Erectile Dysfunction 58, 78, 123
Exhaustion 45
Expectorant 55, 77
Expel Parasites 41
Expels Gas 33, 52, 94
Expels Mucus 33
Expels Mucus & Phlegm 27
Expels Parasites 50
Expels Phlegm 50
Expels Worms 35, 36, 50, 51
External Ulcers 51
External Warts 30
Eye Bacteria 92
Eye diseases 24
Eye Irritation 92
Eye Problems 60
Eyes 33, 58

F

Fat Burning 54
Fatigue 33, 36, 72
Fatty Deposits 53
Female Problems 45, 52
Female Reproductive Glands 47
Female Reproductive System 100
Fever 18, 19, 20, 22, 24, 25, 27, 30, 31, 33, 36, 49, 51, 56, 57, 69, 87, 92, 100, 104, 115, 122
Fever Preventative 28
Flatulence 57
Flu 19, 20, 28, 36, 48, 49, 51, 57, 64, 73, 80, 87, 89, 93, 100
Focus 121
Food Cravings 85
Fractures 43
Free Radical Scavenger 81
Frigidity 45
Fungal Infections 72

G

Gall Bladder 35
Gall Bladder Problems 18

Gall Bladder Support 25, 88
Gallstones 29, 30, 35, 46, 117
Gargle 22, 24, 118
Gas 18, 25, 34, 36, 91, 95, 102
Gastritis 85
Genital Herpes 60, 69, 76
Glandular System Diseases 105
Glandular System Support 20, 24, 72, 104, 105, 108, 117, 119
Goiter 72
Gout 30, 31, 104
Graves' Disease 75
Gum Disease 39, 83
Gum Problems 41

H

Hair Condition (split ends) 67
Hansen's Disease 61
Hardening of the Arteries 63
Hay Fever 31, 91
Headaches 19, 23, 25, 27, 37, 74, 101, 102, 115
Heart Action 107
Heart Disease 72
Heart Disease (Prevention) 102
Heart Function 33
Heart Health 64, 97
Heart Palpitations 63
Heart Protector 59
Heart Stimulant 23
Heart Support 58
Heavy Metal Toxicity 72
Helps Expel Kidney Stones 80
Hemorrhoids 22, 24, 30, 32, 35, 36, 82, 84, 118
Herpes Simplex Virus 66, 69, 75, 76, 79, 87, 88
Hiccups 36
High Blood Pressure 17, 18, 23, 26, 35, 46, 47, 55, 63, 72, 73, 84, 87, 91, 107, 123
HIV 109, 111
Holding Urine 37
Hot Flashes 23, 45, 47
Hyperactivity 65
Hysteria 23

I

Immune System Support 28, 38, 59, 78, 81, 93, 111
Impotence 58, 78, 123
Improves Circulation 36
Incontinence 44, 67, 68
Indigestion 18, 19, 28, 35, 57, 91, 95
Induces Labor 26
Infections 24, 31, 33, 48, 51, 56
Inflamed Joints 56
Inflammation 26, 53, 76, 108, 115, 118, 124
Inflammatory Conditions 89
Insect Bites 19
Insect repellent 94
Insomnia 27, 35, 37, 65, 71, 74, 75, 92, 106, 113
Internal Bleeding 47
Internal Parasites 24
Intestinal Gas 75
Intestinal Health 40
Intestinal System Disorders 52, 60, 76, 110, 124
Intestinal System Support 103, 108
Intestinal Worms 90
Intestines 35
Irritable Bowel Syndrome (IBS) 92, 111

J

Jaundice 18, 28, 30, 33, 35, 120
Joint Inflammation 31

K

Kidney Infections 112
Kidney Problems 21, 23, 29, 31, 33, 63, 67, 68, 80, 102
Kidneys 25
Kidney Stones 68, 80
Kidney Support 80
Kills Bacteria 92
Kills Fungi 92
Kills Molds 92

L

Libido - Lack of 45
Laryngitis 77, 110

Laxative 24, 78, 85, 108, 124
Laxative Action 76
Lead Poisoning 30
Leprosy 61
Liver 120
Liver Conditions 18, 20
Liver Function 60
Liver Health 85, 88, 97
Liver Problems 23, 28, 30, 31, 35, 37, 81, 102
Liver Stimulant 46
Loss of Appetite 57, 64
Low Blood Pressure 107, 123
Lowers Cholesterol 59
Lowers Fever 27
Lung congestion 36
Lung Infections 53, 80
Lung Inflammation 42
Lung Problems 69, 82
Lungs 23, 31
Lung Support 87
Lupus 93
Lymphatic System 120
Lymphatic System Support 31
Lymph Glands 48

M

Malaria 28, 87
Male Problems 45
Male Prostate 105
Measles 28
Memory 25, 32, 58, 78
Memory Loss 61, 101
Menopause 23, 47, 99
Menstrual Cramps 34, 36, 38, 79, 115
Menstrual Problems 23, 25
Menstruation 30, 65
Menstruation (Regulates) 26, 47
Mental and Physical Fatigue 17
Metabolism 47
Migraine Headaches 47
Mild Diuretic 17

Minor Bleeding (Wounds) 22
Miscarriages 117
Morning Sickness 36, 57
Motion Sickness 57, 95
Mouth Infections 70
Mouth Sores 22, 24, 118
Mouth Ulcers 83
Mouthwash 39, 51, 101
Mucus 42
Mumps 28
Muscle Cramps 26, 36
Muscle Spasms 113
Muscular Rheumatism 28

N

Nails 86
Nasal Catarrh 37
Nausea 95
Nephritis 29
Nerves 36
Nervous Conditions 49
Nervous Disorders 23
Nervous Exhaustion 86, 99
Nervous Headaches 36
Nervousness 31
Nervous System Disorders 18, 37, 60, 64, 71, 123
Nervous System Support 26, 27, 47, 52, 61, 65, 74, 75, 86, 92, 99, 101, 106, 109, 117
Neuralgia 26, 37
Nicotine Substitute 77
Nicotine withdrawal 36
Night Blindness 21
Nocturnal Urinary Frequency 98
Normalizes Bowel Function 27
Nose Infections 69
Nose Problems 60
Nourishes the Brain 47

O

Obesity 62, 72, 85
Oral Hygiene 83

Osteoarthritis 87
Osteoporosis 62
Ovarian problems 72
Oxidative Stress 97

P

Pain 23, 36, 115
Pain Killer 39
Pain Relief 93, 113
Pancreas 85
Pancreas Support 33, 56
Parasites 19, 20, 30, 55, 57, 87, 88, 97
Parkinson's Disease 45, 93
Phlebitis 32
Phlegm 53, 66, 110
Pituitary Gland 61
Pituitary Gland Support 17
Pneumonia 42, 49, 77
Pregnancy 84
Pregnancy disorders 26
Premenstrual Syndrome 46, 70
Prevents Heart Disease 102
Prostate Health 68, 97
Prostate Inflammation 98
Prostate Problems 29, 60, 72
Prostate Support 45
Protein Digestion 90
Psoriasis 72, 88, 93
Purifies the Blood 25, 46, 48, 84
Pyorrhea 33, 51

R

Radiation 72
Radiation Therapy 48
Rashes 60
Raynaud's Disease 21
Reduces Fever 17
Reduces Histamine 111
Reduces Inflammation 96
Reduce Sweating from Fever 103
Regulates Menstruation 26, 47

Relaxing 74
Relieves Pain 92
Reproductive Glands 105
Respiratory Infections 19, 25, 95
Respiratory Problems 42
Respiratory System Problems 43
Respiratory System Support 53, 55, 57, 82, 87
Restful Sleep 97
Restlessness 36, 75
Rheumatism 29, 30, 31, 33, 37, 57, 84
Rheumatoid Arthritis 87
Ringworm 24

S

Scalds 118
Schizophrenia, 61
Scurvy 44, 84
Sedative 106, 116, 119
Senility 25
Sensitivity to Light 21
Settles an Upset Stomach 34
Sexual Dysfunction 98
Sexual Energy 45
Sexually Transmitted Diseases 31
Shingles 66
Sinus Infections 95
Skin Conditions 40, 67, 120
Skin diseases 30
Skin Disorders 31
Skin Health 86
Skin Inflammation 38, 93
Skin Irritation 30
Skin Rashes 24
Sleep 65
Smallpox 60
Snake Bites 19
Sore Muscles 118
Sores 43
Sore Throat 20, 22, 26, 28, 33, 51, 53, 82, 83, 110, 114, 118
Sore Throat (Gargle) 95
Spasms 26, 34, 36

Spleen 35, 120
Spleen Function 60
Spleen Support 25, 56
Stamina 121
Stimulates Appetite 17
Stings 48
Stomach Problems 43, 60
Stomach Support 56
Stomach Ulcers 38, 40, 111
Stomach Upset 75, 95
Stops Bleeding 30
Strengthen Bones 67
Strengthens the Heart 25
Strengthens the Lungs 25
Strengthen Teeth 67
Stress 36, 59, 74, 76, 92, 106
Stroke 33, 58
Structural System Support 43
Sugar Cravings 62
Supports the Immune System 21
Swollen Joints 49
Swollen Lymph Nodes 55
Syphilis 104

T

Throat Gargle 38
Throat Infections 69, 70
Throat Problems 60
Thyroid Function 24
Thyroid Problems 72, 75
Tinnitus 58
Tonic 17, 28, 43, 47
Tonsillitis 24
Toothache 34, 41
Tooth Decay 83
Toxic Waste Removal 53, 96, 124
Tranquilizer 27, 106, 116
Triglyceride Levels 62
Tumor Fighter 33, 39
Tumors 24, 48, 68, 93, 114

U

Ulcerative Colitis 111
Ulcers 33, 72, 93, 114
Ulcers (Internal & External) 43
Upset Stomach 22, 36
Urinary System Disorders 17, 62, 64, 67
Urinary System Disorders (Men) 98, 105
Urinary System Support 70, 87, 112
Urinary Tract Infections 29, 44, 67, 68, 70, 88, 91, 103
Urinary Tract Inflammation 112
Uterine Bleeding 84
Uterine Cramps 34
Uterine Problems 23, 26

V

Vaginal Problems 60
Vaginitis 26
Varicose Veins 21, 32, 33, 58, 61
Vertigo 58
Virus 28, 55, 110
Vision Problems 92
Vomiting 36, 75

W

Waste Elimination 83
Water Retention 37
Weak Arteries 46
Weight Loss 37, 46, 54, 85, 121
Weight Loss Programs 123
Weight Management 62
Whooping Cough 19, 110
Worms 19, 24, 28, 30, 57, 64, 89, 97
Wound Healing 22, 24, 31, 33, 38, 43, 48, 51, 53, 60, 66, 83, 103, 107, 108, 109, 110, 112, 119

Y

Yeast Infections 55, 70

Index of Herbs

A

Alfalfa 17

B

Barberry 18
Basil 19
Bayberry 20
Bilberry 21
Blackberry 22
Black Cohosh 23
Black Walnut 24
Blessed Thistle 25
Blue Cohosh 26
Blue Vervain 27
Boneset 28
Buchu 29
Buckthorn 30
Burdock 31
Butchers Broom 32

C

Capsicum 33
Caraway 34
Cascara Sagrada 35
Catnip 36
Cats Claw (Una de Gato 111
Celery 37
Chamomile 38
Chaparral 39
Chickweed 40
Cloves 41
Coltsfoot 42
Comfrey 43
Cranberry 44

D

Damiana 45
Dandelion 46
Dong Quai 47

E

Echinacea 48
Elderflower 49
Elecampane 50
Eucalyptus 51

F

Fennel 52
Fenugreek 53

G

Garcinia Cambogia 54
Garlic 55
Gentian 56
Ginger 57
Ginkgo Biloba 58
Ginseng 59
Golden Seal 60
Gotu Kola 61

H

Hawthorn 63
Hibiscus 64
Hops 65
Horehound 66
Horsetail 67
Hydrangea 68
Hyssop 69

J

Juniper 70

K

Kava Kava 71
Kelp 72
Kudzu 73

L

Lavender 74
Lemon Balm 75
Licorice 76
Lobelia 77

M

Maca 78
Marjoram 79
Marshmallow 80
Milk Thistle 81
Mullein 82
Myrrh 83

N

Nettle 84
Nopal 85

O

Oatstraw 86
Olive Leaf 87
Oregano 89
Oregon Grape 88

P

Papaya 90
Parsley 91
Passion Flower 92
Pau D'Arco 93
Pennyroyal 94
Peppermint 95
Psyllium 96
Pumpkin 97
Pygeum 98

R

Red Clover 99
Red Raspberry 100
Rosemary 101

S

Saffron 102
Sage 103
Sarsaparilla 104
Saw Palmetto 105
Shepherds Purse 107
Skullcap 106
Slippery Elm 108
St. John's Wort 109

T

Thyme 110

U

Una de Gato (Cats Claw) 111
Uva Ursi 112

V

Valerian 113
Violet 114

W

White Willow 115
Wild Cherry 116
Wild Yam 117
Witch Hazel 118

Y

Yarrow 119
Yellow Dock 120
Yerba Mate 121
Yerba Santa 122
Yohimbe 123
Yucca 124

www.ingramcontent.com/pod-product-compliance
Lightning Source LLC
Chambersburg PA
CBHW070659290526
45790CB00001B/386